KAREN AMEN'S
THE
Bottom
Line

Also by Karen Amen

The Crunch
(with Tee Dobinson)

KAREN AMEN'S
THE
Bottom Line

THE NEW AND DYNAMIC WAY TO TIGHTEN AND TONE THE BUTTOCKS AND THIGHS

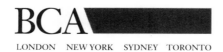

LONDON   NEW YORK   SYDNEY   TORONTO

This edition published in 1996
by BCA by arrangement with Vermilion
an imprint of Ebury Press

CN 2784

Printed and bound in Great Britain by
Butler & Tanner Ltd, Frome and London

CREDITS

Edited by Jan Bowmer
Designed by Roger Walker/Graham Harmer
Cover designed by Jerry Goldie
Cover modelled by Karen Amen
Nutritional advice by Andrea Rizzo
Exercises demonstrated by Karen Amen, Peter Beuner, Jess Kleiderman,
Luis Perez, Andrea Rizzo and Michael Stevens
Cover photographs by Roberto Rabanne
Inside photographs by Randy O'Rourke and Roberto Rabanne
Illustrations by Leslie Dean
Outfits courtesy of Everlast, Converse and Amen's Actionwear
Trainers courtesy of Reebok International

CONTENTS

ACKNOWLEDGEMENTS

Nancy, Lou and my sisses – the crew. Could not have made it without your love and support.

Carol. Cannot wait for the opportunity to be your crutch. Thanks for holding me up. Much love.

All my clients. Thank you for your patience and support. I have been so lucky in my life in always having the best to work with – you guys are the best!

The staff at the Reebok Sports Club/NY. Thanks for your kind words, motivation and encouragement.

Jessica, Fred, Randy and Bertha. You literally pulled me through to the end. Thanks.

Jan. What can I say? I hope to work with you on many more projects. More importantly, I hope that our friendship lasts a very long time. Thanks.

One group of people, many of whom I have not yet had the opportunity to meet but hope to at some point in my life – the readers. Thanks for letting me know that the programs work for you and help you to attain your goals. Health and Happiness.

Karen

ABOUT THE AUTHOR

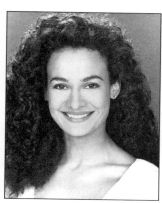

Karen Amen has been training fitness professionals, celebrities and the general public for over a decade and, since 1985, has been involved in the qualification and continuing education of thousands of instructors and trainers worldwide. A former gold medallist in the US National Aerobics Championships, she brings diverse disciplines with her into the fitness arena.

Karen is a popular presenter of lifestyle and fitness programs on the NBC, Fox TV and Via Com television networks in the US. Operating out of New York City, she currently spends much of her time working with people with special needs, keeping them fit, helping them to maintain a positive lifestyle and, in some cases, helping people cope with serious illness. She also trains and teaches classes at the Reebok Sports Club/NY.

Her first book, *The Crunch*, was an instant bestseller and has been published in four languages. The video based on the book has won several awards, including an award for the best instructional video of 1995.

Introduction

Would you like to have firmer buttocks and leaner thighs?
Would you like to have more shapely legs, tighten those outer thighs and
achieve a sleek, more streamlined look? Or are you simply tired of the old
traditional floor exercises and are ready for something new? Then read on.

If you're unhappy with the size or shape of your buttocks, legs and thighs,
don't worry. You *can* do something about it. That's why I've written this book,
so that you and the thousands of women – and, yes, men too – out there can
help yourselves by applying the training methods that I have used
successfully with thousands of private clients and fitness professionals over
the last decade.

The lower body is much more of a problem area for women than men.
Women tend to have a larger percentage of sex-specific fat in this area, along
with a wider pelvis for child-bearing. That's why it's extremely important for
women to watch the amount of fat in their diet as well as to follow a specific
exercise plan. This is where my Bottom Line program comes in. We don't
have to give into Nature's ageing process. As we get older, it is possible for us
to fight the natural tendency of sagging rears and floppy legs with a solid
training program. In this book I am going to give you the ammunition you
need through a series of exercises that will provide you with a practical and
effective solution.

But I've got wide hips and my thighs are really enormous!

So, can I *really* tighten and tone my buttocks and thighs, I hear you ask? Of
course you can, and this new and dynamic muscle-shaping program will help
you achieve just that – safely, accurately and effectively. Whatever your age,
shape, body type or level of fitness, whether you have short legs or wide hips,
have or have not been exercising for some time, as long as your general
health is good, this program will provide you with the necessary tools to
achieve those goals. All you have to do is follow the step-by-step instructions
and you'll learn how to use the muscles of the legs effectively, how to firm
them up and improve their overall shape without adding unsightly bulk.

And there's more. This program will also help improve your posture and alignment and enhance your ability to perform everyday tasks such as walking, lifting, sitting and standing properly or to bounce back after a fall, avoiding serious injury. You'll gain increased physical strength, flexibility, control and balance, all of which can help slow down the ageing process. Once you start to shape up and become stronger, your new-found poise will bring you heaps of confidence – you'll feel more attractive, sexier and more vibrant. Believe me, I see this transformation all the time with my clients. The women start to wear skirts more often or find they can now slip into the snugly fitting trousers they have longed to wear for some time. After just two to three weeks of training, they turn up for their exercise session *without* the huge sweatshirts that they once used to don to cover up their bodies. The men start to wear bike shorts to train in and tuck their T-shirts into their shorts, instead of letting them loosely hang out as a form of camouflage. It is these small changes that make me realize how successful my methods have been in empowering my clients to adopt a more positive attitude toward their bodies and helping them to understand that they have more control over the shape of their bodies than they ever imagined.

Will I be healthier?

To ensure that you achieve – and maintain – the maximum benefits and to complete the formula for health and wellbeing, it is important to look at your lifestyle habits as a whole. Toning and strengthening exercises can have a dramatic effect on the overall shape of your legs. What I want is for you to have the best body you can possibly achieve, and specific exercise is just part of the equation. For optimum health benefits, therefore, you'll need to eat the right kind of foods, in the right proportions – and I've got some great eating tips for you in chapter 5 – as well as adding some form of aerobic activity to your program. Choose something convenient and enjoyable such as walking, jogging or swimming and try to practise three to five times a week. As long as you are able to sustain it for 15–30 minutes without stopping, any one of these activities can increase the strength of your heart and lungs and, together with this Bottom Line program and a sensible eating plan, can put you on the right path to a healthier, more fulfilling lifestyle. This equation would not be complete without regular medical check-ups.

Will I lose weight?

Toning and strengthening exercise helps us to maintain and increase our muscle mass. Since the actual chemical process by which fat and sugar is broken down in the body takes place in the muscle tissue, if we increase the density of our muscle tissue by doing specific strength training, then we will also increase the number of sites in the body where calories are used up. Hence, we become more efficient at calorie-burning. Aerobic activity also burns calories, so don't forget to include this in your program.

If you are overweight, then you'll also need to reduce your calorie intake, so do check out the healthy eating guidelines in chapter 5. However, combining a sensible eating plan with toning and strengthening, as well as regular aerobic exercise, will ensure that any weight you lose is fat, not muscle. Muscle tissue is more taut and compact than fat tissue and therefore takes up less space. By increasing your muscle tissue you can actually drop down a dress size or two. So don't worry about the scales, just focus on your dress size.

Since both our metabolic rate – that's the rate at which we burn calories – and the amount of muscle tissue we have decrease with age, exercise along with healthy eating and a positive lifestyle attitude can have a measurable impact on slowing down the ageing process and improve self-confidence at any age.

But I've not exercised for ages

If you are new to exercising, then you've chosen a great place to start. Frequently, I am asked by women if it is possible to change the shape of their legs, even if they have never exercised before or, at least, not exercised for some time. My answer is, sure you can! If you have not worked out before or have not worked out for a while, just have a little patience. In fact, to begin with, your rate of improvement will actually be greater than someone who works out regularly. Once you start to exercise on a regular basis and once you have achieved your initial goal, over time, your rate of improvement will slow down. But then, it won't take so much effort to maintain it. It is *never* too late to begin exercising and make a positive improvement to your body shape and your health.

I already work out regularly, so what's in it for me?

If you already work out regularly, you'll discover some new and exciting ideas for floor work as well as some interesting variations on old favourites. So, if you're tired of your old floor routine and are ready for some new challenges, this book is also for you.

What about men?

Although the majority of those who want to change the shape of their lower bodies tend to be women, men, too, can benefit from this program. As they age, men tend to lose strength and firmness in their legs and can also suffer from constant back problems, in part due to decreased flexibility in the back of the legs. Once they are no longer playing the sports they so frequently practised at school, men often find that their buttocks begin to get 'soft' and that the leg muscles are not as strong and firm as they used to be. This, combined with the subsequent decrease in flexibility, can create real problems, particularly with respect to the low back.

Some of the exercises in this book are based on conditioning drills that are commonly used in preparation for sports participation, while in other exercises the positioning of the body can render the moves quite challenging. Many of the exercises are designed to take the legs through their full range of motion, and this, together with the flexibility section in this book, can greatly increase suppleness in the back of the legs and in the low back, improving overall leg and torso strength.

In my classes, around 40–50 per cent of the students are male, and all have commented on how challenging they find the exercises. In fact, many of their wives have also thanked me for the changes I have effected in their husbands. At first, I was a little puzzled by what they meant. One wife, noting my confusion, explained that her husband's quality of movement had greatly improved and he no longer complained of back discomfort 'at the most inappropriate of moments', as she put it, which in turn greatly improved the quality of *her* life. I have to admit, I chuckled a bit. And the plain truth is, men, that we women also like to see firm, tight legs and buttocks on our men. Did you really think we didn't?

So, can anyone benefit?

Whatever your current fitness level or ability, whether you're male or female, here you'll find a truly effective and balanced program to sculpt your lower body – a program that will not only shape and define your muscles but that will also improve your overall appearance and health, increase your confidence, poise and energy levels and fight the ageing process. That's the bottom line.

CHAPTER ONE

So, what's different about this program?

When I started to write this book I looked up the word 'program' in the dictionary. Here is what I found: 'An organized effort to achieve a goal by stages'. This is the exact philosophy of the Bottom Line program, and I want *you* to work through the program with this in mind.

Here, I have devised four easy-to-follow but progressively challenging workout plans, designed to produce a balanced muscle development and target common misalignment habits while reshaping your bottom half with the minimum risk of injury. Throughout, I've used visual imagery and created tips which will enable you to find the appropriate body positioning for your particular body type.

This program requires no special equipment, but for extra variety or to provide support, I have incorporated the use of a few household items. These items include a simple broomstick, a chair, a beach ball and a wooden box or step – or you can even use the stairs in your home. For those of you with a resistance band or tubing, I have included an exercise to show how you can incorporate this into your training. However, this exercise can also be done without the tubing or band and still prove very effective.

The muscles of the lower body, along with the abdominal and back muscles, are instrumental in helping us to acquire a balanced, well-proportioned body and, consequently, to maintain a proper posture and muscular balance. That's why one of the chief focuses throughout this book is on proper technique and body placement so that you can begin immediately to hold the body in a more correct alignment, not just when exercising but also at all other times of the day.

To this end, in some of the exercises, I have included photographs that illustrate the *incorrect* body positioning. These serve to highlight the typical errors that we all make – and I see these often, when teaching classes or working with clients on a one-to-one basis. Incorrect positioning can lead to discomfort in the joints and even enforce some of the muscular imbalances which we are trying to correct in this program.

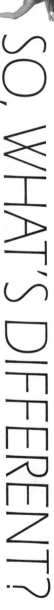

SO, WHAT'S DIFFERENT?

Look carefully at these 'wrong' photographs to ensure that you avoid these common pitfalls. Proper positioning is the key to achieving your best possible shape, ensuring that every single repetition counts toward improving your physical shape and strength. After all, one of the most common excuses for not exercising regularly is lack of time. Ensuring that you acquire the proper positioning in all these exercises means you'll be able to maximize your efforts while minimizing the amount of time you spend on each workout.

TRADITIONAL FLOOR WORK VERSUS A MORE DYNAMIC METHOD OF TRAINING

If you are familiar with the traditional lower body exercises – you know, the ones where you lie on the floor and move your legs out to the side or up and down, you'll notice that we have adapted many of these by changing the positioning. Furthermore, this program includes a lot of standing leg work. So what's the reason for this?

The fitter and stronger we are, the better we are able to perform everyday activities such as walking, sitting or standing properly and for longer, shifting our body weight around, or lifting and balancing as we reach for objects. So, in this program we concentrate on what I call functional floor work – floor work that takes place primarily in the standing position, with and without additional external support. You'll learn to use your abdomen as your constant source of support.

Unlike many traditional leg toning exercises where you lie on the floor in a horizontal position and perform a number of repetitions of a single movement, the exercises in this book are specifically designed to mimic the actions and body mechanics that we use in everyday life and also to work against the pull of gravity. The kind of movements that we perform in the 'lying down horizontal-type exercises' seldom apply to 'real' life. And when we do lie down in 'real' life we are usually resting in a reclined position. Generally, it's when we wish to stand up that the ability to push our body weight around against the pull of gravity becomes more useful. However, in this program I have also included some interesting variations on conventional leg exercises which place specific muscle groups in a position where the resistance against gravity is greater.

Stay active, be functional – and defy gravity

Over the years, my experience in fitness has taught me something I would like to share with you. Those individuals, including myself, who have not only exercised on a regular basis but, more importantly, have also made continuous and correct use of their muscles to stand, sit and walk properly, have bodies which remain firm and extremely functional and which seem to defy the ageing process. You would not believe how active some of my senior clients are – and by senior I mean 80 years and above – and how their active and functional bodies enable them to live incredibly full lifestyles. Their bodies are literally defying the long-term effects of gravity.

Reap optimum benefits

Bearing in mind the importance of functional-type exercise, many of the individual exercises in this program target many muscle groups simultaneously, enabling the muscles to work in the way that we need them to perform on a daily basis. For instance, when we walk, run or get up from a sitting position, it is the combined action of a number of muscle groups that enables us to perform these activities. The individual strength of each muscle group is important, but equally important is their relative strength to each other.

These exercises will not only shape up and strengthen your legs and buttocks but also improve your sense of balance and your ability to perform sports. What's more, weight-bearing exercises, such as standing floor work and exercises that involve jumping or springing off the floor, help increase bone density, which in turn can help prevent the onset of the brittle bone condition known as osteoporosis.

Maximize your efforts

Once you're familiar with the basic technique in this program, we will start to introduce 'travelling' moves. Here, the aim is to complete a sequence of movements in a fluid, dynamic and controlled fashion, enabling you to contract (tighten) the muscles at the beginning and also throughout the exercise, rather than just hitting a single position over and over again as in a traditional toning exercise where we generally contract the muscles only at the end of the movement.

With certain types of training, each time we work our muscles, waste products are produced within the muscle fibres. In conventional toning exercises, because the actual working phase of the exercise is generally concentrated at the end of the movement, the overall range of movement in

7

SO, WHAT'S DIFFERENT?

the exercise is small. This encourages a more rapid build-up of waste products, specifically lactic acid, which diminishes your capacity to contract a muscle and therefore minimizes your efforts.

For instance, if you were lying on your side and performing a number of leg raises, while maintaining the proper leg position with the knee facing forward, you might begin to feel an uncomfortable burning sensation in the outer thigh muscle being worked and feel unable to continue lifting the leg. This discomfort is due to the build-up of lactic acid in the outer thigh muscle which can lead to premature muscle fatigue and slow down your rate of progress.

With travelling moves, however, we work in a greater range of motion, which helps prevent such a rapid formation of lactic acid, thereby delaying the feeling of discomfort and enabling you to complete more repetitions. At the same time, the greater range of motion enables a greater number of muscle fibres to be recruited which encourages the muscles to become firmer and stronger and results in a more complete and overall training for your bottom line.

Avoid a 'bulky' look

There is a further advantage in the type of exercises I have put together for you in this program. The use of short-range movements in conventional toning exercises means that certain muscle fibres are utilized over and over again which, unless you are a very tall, long-boned individual, encourages the development of bulk. However, in this program, we will be focusing on long-range movements that bring about a muscle contraction at the beginning and throughout the full range of movement, which leads to firm, lean and shapely legs without a bulky look. Most women would agree that they want firm, strong, lean-looking legs, and the methods in this program are designed to help you accomplish just that.

THE BOTTOM LINE BENEFITS

If you apply yourself to this program and practise regularly and consistently, here are some of the benefits you can expect:

▶ firmer buttocks
▶ more shapely legs
▶ improved overall body shape
▶ increased poise and confidence

▶ improved balance

▶ fewer low-back problems

▶ increased control and strength

▶ greater flexibility

▶ improved ability to carry out everyday tasks

▶ reduced risk of joint injuries

▶ increased energy levels

▶ more efficient use of calories

▶ enhanced potential for your muscles to fight the effects of gravity

▶ improved bone density.

Sounds good? Then let's find out more.

SO, WHAT'S DIFFERENT?

9

CHAPTER TWO

Perfect poise: a body in balance

Good posture and alignment are fundamental to the success of this program. So, let's start out with an overview of how to stand and sit properly using the leg muscles. Once you know how the various muscles interplay to effect good postural alignment and how this relates to the mechanics of the Bottom Line program, you'll be ready to move on to the plans themselves.

More and more people are beginning to realize that good posture is desirable not only from an aesthetic point of view – people with good poise always attract our attention – but that it is also an indication of our overall health and wellbeing. It aids our natural breathing pattern, helps protect our internal organs and structures from damage and reduces our risk of suffering low-back problems.

We'd all like to look and feel younger, be stronger and possess the ease of movement and sense of balance that is normally associated with youth. Maintaining a good and balanced posture enables us to function better and improves our ability to perform everyday tasks. It ensures that the body's structures are better equipped to brave the wear and tear of everyday use and help fight the onslaught of the ageing process – and, in some cases, even slow it down.

That's why in this Bottom Line program, as well as in my earlier Crunch program, I stress the connection between attaining your desired body shape and the importance of proper posture and daily body maintenance. Let's face it, the body is a mechanical entity – a highly complex and fascinating machine. In this program I have brought you the latest and safest methods that will help you get your body into its best possible shape and enable it to function at peak efficiency.

WHAT IS A BODY IN BALANCE?

When we stand in a balanced posture, no one structure of the legs or back has to work disproportionately harder than another. The head is balanced between the shoulders and the chin is not jutting forward. Shoulders are back and down and the abdomen is lifted. The weight is distributed evenly through the legs right through to the bottom of the feet, and the hips, knees and ankles are lined up. This allows the natural curves of the spine to be in a healthy relationship with one another – a relationship which enables a greater ease of movement and allows the internal structures their proper space. Think of this as your Torso neutral – or T-neutral – position.

The bones in our limbs are not directly connected to each other but are separated by joints. If we didn't have joints, we would not be able to bend our arms or legs and we'd move in a completely different way! A good alignment generally allows us to maintain an even pressure throughout the joints which helps prevent some of the body's structures wearing away at a much faster rate than others.

There are two extremely common misalignment problems over which most of us have control. The first is standing with knees hyperextended – in other words, standing with the knees pressed back so that the knee joints are locked. The second is asymmetrical standing, where the body weight is shifted to one side – and most of us have a preferred side of the body which bears the brunt of our weight.

Take a good look at the photographs (right) which illustrate how hyperextension of the knees can, over time, overstretch the internal structures in the back of the knees, minimize the use of your front thigh muscles and buttocks and cause the buttock muscles to become slack through underuse.

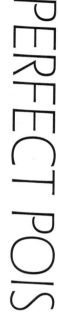

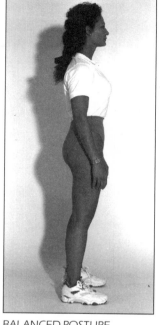

BALANCED POSTURE

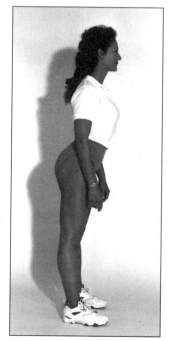

IMBALANCED POSTURE

1 1

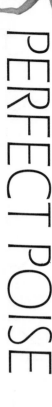

PERFECT POISE

Standing with our weight on one side greatly increases the pressure placed on the joints on the side of the body where we are placing our weight. If we continue to lock the knees or stand with the weight over to one side, a disproportionate pressure is constantly being placed on the internal structures of the hip, knee and ankle joints. Over time, this can result in a number of joint and bone disorders which greatly weaken the joints.

One extremely common disorder with which most of us are familiar is Dowager's hump, an extreme forward curve of the upper back. The sufferer actually develops a hump in the back which can eventually prevent them from standing upright. Although in some people this disorder may be caused by a specific disease, in many cases it is the consequence of a lifetime of hunching over.

In the case of teenagers, constant standing with the weight over to one side of the body can contribute to scoliosis, an abnormal curvature of the spine where the spine curves sideways to form a 'C' or 'S' shape. The symptoms are varied and can range from mild discomfort on the one hand to more severe ones which are serious enough to warrant full body traction.

Of course, there are other reasons why some people may develop these disorders, but we do know that standing incorrectly can have long-term damaging effects on our functional abilities.

THE IMPORTANCE OF MUSCULAR BALANCE

Some of the muscles in the body are quite naturally stronger than others. For instance, have you ever heard of anyone tearing their quadricep (front thigh) muscles? No. Yet how often have you known someone to injure the opposing hamstring muscles at the back of the thighs? Many times, I expect. The front thigh muscles, quite naturally, tend to be 33 per cent stronger than the hamstrings. So, it's particularly important to pay attention to the hamstring muscles and ensure they receive adequate strengthening and flexibility work.

If we overuse or overtrain certain muscles at the expense of others, then we can upset the natural balance of strength and flexibility. When the opposing muscle groups that surround any given joint have relatively good strength and flexibility, the internal pressure of that particular joint is fairly even throughout. However, if one muscle group is too tight or lacking in muscle tone, this disrupts the pressure inside the joint and leads to what is known as a muscular imbalance, which greatly increases the risk of injury.

For instance, if you were to constantly stand with shoulders slumped forward, over time, the front of the shoulders would become less flexible and the shoulder joints would shift forward slightly, greatly weakening the upper back. To rectify this, you would need to do a great deal of work that involved opening the chest and shoulder area.

A relative balance between the muscles is therefore necessary if we are to avoid any kind of joint or back problem.

THE MUSCLES WE WILL BE TARGETING

Many of the muscles in the legs attach to the pelvic and low-back region, which is why, along with the abdominal and back muscles, they are responsible for maintaining good posture.

Here are the primary muscle groups we will be concentrating on, together with a brief description of their functions in terms of this Bottom Line program. You will see that, often, more than one muscle group is responsible for a specific action.

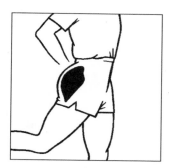

Gluteals (buttocks)

Functions

Hip extension (illustrated). Opening the hip at the top of the thigh by moving the thigh bone backward, away from the front of the body. For example, it is the position of a runner's back leg as he or she places the back leg on the starting block.

Abduction. Moving the leg out to the side, away from the centre of the body.

Outward rotation. Moving the thigh muscle around a centre point, for instance, when we turn the leg out.

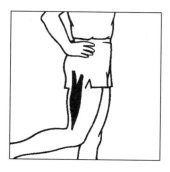

Hamstrings (back of thighs)

Functions

Hip extension. Opening the hip at the top of the thigh by moving the thigh bone backward, away from the front of the body.

Outward rotation. Moving the thigh muscle around a centre point.

Knee flexion (illustrated). Bending the knee, particularly when the thigh bone moves backward.

1 3

PERFECT POISE

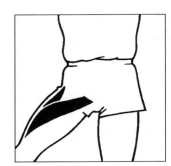

Abductors (outer thighs)

Function

Abduction. Moving the leg out to the side, away from the centre of the body.

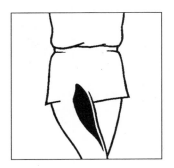

Adductors (inner thighs)

Function

Adduction. Moving the leg sideways, toward the centre of the body, allowing the leg to cross either in front of or behind the other leg.

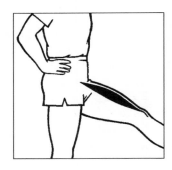

Quadriceps (front of thighs)

Functions

Hip flexion. Bending the hip, for instance, when we kick the leg up.

Knee extension. Straightening the knee.

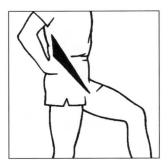

Hip Flexors (top of thighs)

Function

Hip flexion. Bending the leg at the hip, for instance, when we kick the leg up.

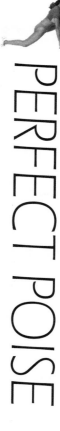

TEN TIPS FOR PROPER TECHNIQUE

1 In the standing position, always keep your upper body lifted.

2 Always try to align the shoulders above the hips, hips above the knees and knees above the ankles.

3 In moves where one leg is in front of or behind the other, avoid leaning forward. Instead, keep the upper body lifted directly above the hips.

4 When performing rotational movements (turning the legs outward), ensure that the turn-out action comes from rotating the hips at the top of the thighs and not by pushing the knees outward. The knees should follow the direction of the hips, and the ankles and toes should follow the direction of the knees. Think 'hips, knees, ankles' – in this order.

5 When descending into a squat, lunge or similar movement try not to let the knees wobble.

6 When using any form of support, such as a broomstick or chair, try not to hang onto it with your full body weight. Instead, think of lifting away from the support. This is where your abdomen comes into play.

7 When moving the leg backward as in a hip extension, be sure to really pull up with your abdomen to keep the movement out of your low back and confined to the hip joint.

8 Maintaining a constant lift in the abdomen will greatly assist you to keep your balance.

9 Start each exercise by contracting (tightening) the muscles and try to maintain this contraction throughout the full range of movement.

10 Believe in yourself. Thinking strong will make you strong.

PERFECT POISE

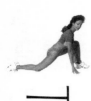

CHAPTER THREE

The Bottom Line Program

HOW IT WORKS

The four plans in this book together form a progressive, step-by-step program that will make a real difference to your bottom line. Each plan in itself forms a self-contained workout that focuses on the development of specific skills to firm and tone the leg muscles. Start with Plan One and work your way through each plan at your own pace, only moving up to the next plan when you are proficient in the skills of the current plan. Remember, with this program you are going to make an organized effort to achieve your goal in *stages*. So, think of each plan as a stage or link in a chain. As you progress through the plans you will add further links to your chain that will lead you to your ultimate goal of strong, shapely legs and improved posture.

Plan One: Lean Technique

Here's where we learn the basic positioning and placement, the first link in our chain and an essential one if you are to complete the program effectively. This plan lays down the foundations on which all the following plans are based and provides you with all the information you need on where you should place your head, shoulders, hips, knees and ankles in relation to each other, in a variety of positions that we'll be using in the later plans. Taking time to master the proper technique and correct body positioning will help you maximize the benefits of your workout while minimizing the amount of time spent exercising.

Plan Two: Striking a Balance

Next, we are going to cultivate our sense of balance, by utilizing the muscles of the abdomen, back and legs. We will also begin to introduce travelling moves into the program so that you really begin to execute each exercise in a more dynamic fashion – another step toward firmer buttocks and leaner legs.

Plan Three: Changing Tactics

Here, we're going to combine some traditional horizontal floor work with unsupported standing work that involves some longer sequences of movement to challenge your sense of balance further, adding more links to our chain and climbing further toward that goal.

Plan Four: Right on Target

This plan is going to challenge your range of motion further by introducing some springs, leaps and sports-type movements into your program – the final link in our chain. You'll be really springing into your best possible shape, while increasing your energy level. It's goodbye to the jiggles!

GETTING THE MOST OUT OF THIS PROGRAM

Whatever your ability, always start with Plan One to make sure you are familiar with the basics and can complete the maximum number of repetitions in proper form before you move on to the more challenging exercises. So, even if you have been exercising regularly for years, take time to recap on your basic technique.

If you're new to exercising, you'll need to take a little longer to familiarize yourself with the basics in Plan One. Take it slowly and don't worry if you can't achieve the suggested number of repetitions at first. Just do as many as you can, really concentrating on finding your correct positioning, then gradually increase the number of repetitions as you become stronger. If you don't challenge your body, you can't expect to change it. Remember, it's not a race, the only person you are competing against is yourself.

Practice makes perfect

If you have not been able to exercise for a year or so, aim to practise Plan One twice a week, on non-consecutive days. Once you can get through Plan One, completing all the recommended repetitions in proper form, you can increase to three times a week or move on to the next plan.

If you are a regular exerciser, aim to practise Plan One three times a week, again on non-consecutive days. Once you can complete the recommended

1 7

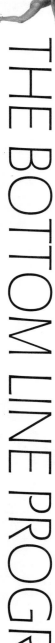

repetitions in proper form and feel confident with each move, you can progress to the next plan.

Continue like this with each of the plans, making sure you have fully mastered all the moves before you step up a plan. If at any time you take a break from the program or are inconsistent with your practice, always start with the previous plan when you rejoin the program, and work up from there.

If you are feeling really confident and wish to practise more frequently, that's fine. But be sure not to work out using the same plan on two consecutive days in order to allow sufficient recovery times for the muscles. Muscles do need some rest, especially if they've been worked hard. This allows them time for repair and to get used to the new demands that are being made on them. Ensuring you allow sufficient recuperation time for the muscles will lead to enhanced results and minimize the risk of injury.

It's not how much you do, it's how you do it

It's not the quantity of repetitions but the quality of each repetition that counts, which is why this program is so time-efficient. It's far better to do 16 repetitions in good form than to attempt 20 or 30 in an unapplied and undisciplined fashion so that only five or ten of these repetitions are really effective. So aim to gradually build up the number each time you work out. The determining factor as to whether you should add another set of repetitions is whether you can do the prescribed amount with strength and proper form. To make genuine progress, you will have to be prepared to work out of your comfort zone just a little in order to provide sufficient challenge for the muscles. If you always stay within your comfort zone, your body is not forced to make any adaptations. Hence, it will never progress to the point where it could and should be.

Get into gear for exercise

Always start your workout by gearing up and preparing your joints and muscles for exercise (see pages 21–32). Getting the mind and body into gear for exercise is an essential part of the process. Try not to neglect this section of the program as it will increase the effectiveness of your Bottom Line workout. Likewise, at the end of your exercise session, take some time to wind down and work on improving your flexibility (see pages 81–94). At this stage your body will be nice and warm and more receptive to the stretches in this section of the program.

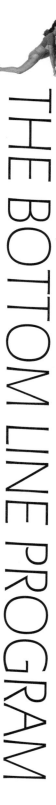

Stay committed and consistent

Commitment and consistency are important if you are to see genuine results. So, formulate a plan where you set aside a period of 10–20 minutes on two or three days each week to practise this program – and aim to *stick* to that plan. It's a good idea to set certain time slots so that you know that at seven o'clock on Monday the next 20 minutes will be for you. Of course, there will occasionally be times when you may have to skip your training session on a particular day. That's OK. Life is like that. Just make doubly sure you do your workout on the next day and mentally re-affirm your goals. Remember why you picked up this book in the first place? You want to make improvements to your body shape. So, go for it! Focus on the numerous benefits you will achieve. I'm convinced that once you start this Bottom Line program you'll find it so challenging and the results will be so rewarding that you'll be totally committed.

Visualize your goals

Set yourself some goals, then visualize them! Make them specific – you want stronger legs, tighter thighs. You have chosen to pick up this book because you want a leaner, stronger body – so make it happen! Spend time actually thinking about how good you'll feel and how much tighter your legs are going to be. Imagine your body becoming tighter, more toned and stronger each day and feel your confidence growing. You *are* going to achieve a tight, toned sleek body. Picture yourself succeeding. Life can be so much easier when we think positive rather than dwelling on the negative. We can be quite good at putting ourselves down – some of us have spent a lifetime doing it. Now, you're going to change all that. Think it, and you'll be it! Remember, I'll be with you every step of the way.

Record your progress

To encourage you to continue and inspire you on to greater goals, keep a record of your progress. Make a copy of the Training Log on page 119 and fill this in after every workout. Stick this in a highly visible place, such as on the door of your refrigerator, so that you have a constant reminder of your daily accomplishments. Make a note of any improvements you see and feel, and keep a note of any other activities or exercise you undertake. Likewise, keep a record of your eating habits, using the Food Diary on page 120, and note down any changes you make. It's been proven time and time again that by

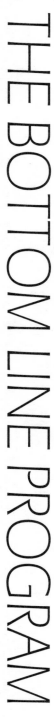

THE BOTTOM LINE PROGRAM

recording your progress in this way, you are more likely to be consistently successful in achieving your goals.

Keep progressing

Once you have completed all four plans successfully, you can interchange them as you wish or move on to the Bottom Line Break in chapter 4. Here, you'll find a number of suggestions for changing the way you stimulate your muscles to ensure that ongoing progress can be made and to add further variety and challenge to your program. This will prevent you from reaching a plateau and enable you to see continuous changes. In this section, you'll also find some great new ideas for partner work to provide extra motivation and incentive for your workout.

This is your program, so make it work for you. Remember, should you find your technique slipping, or if you just feel your movements are incorrect and you need to recap on the basics, return to Plan One to give yourself a refresher course.

A word of warning

This program is intended for people in good health. If you have ever suffered a hip, back or knee problem or have not had a medical check-up for over a year, it is essential you obtain your doctor's clearance before commencing this program.

If you should feel any sharp or sudden pain or dizziness while practising these or any other exercises, stop immediately and, if necessary, seek the appropriate medical advice.

GEARING UP

OK, armed with the basics on how the muscles of the legs work, you are ready for first gear – the warm-up or preparatory movements. You've gotten this far in the book, so it's obvious that you are committed to training your body. You want to feel better, stronger, more confident about your body, and this preparatory session is the first step toward these aims.

Let's start by preparing ourselves mentally. Before you picked up this book to begin your workout, odds are your mind was elsewhere. You may have just come home from work or just got the children off to school, or perhaps you're taking a break in the middle of your busy day. You want to have a good training session, one that achieves results? Well, then your mind needs to concentrate on what you are about to undertake and the benefits you are going to achieve. This is your time and you deserve to have a little time to invest in your health and wellbeing.

This series of movements is designed to warm you up and prepare your joints for the exercises that follow. In this section we are not looking to add any resistance yet, but just aiming to raise the temperature of the body and muscles and take the joints through similar movements to those they will be undertaking with more resistance later on.

Move fluidly through each movement *without force*, using as full a range of motion as possible and gently increasing your range with each repetition. This will serve to oil up the joints and prepare them for the stresses we are going to place them under. Research has shown that preparing the joints and warming the muscles in this way increases the actual number of muscle fibres that can be pulled into action in the toning exercises themselves, thereby increasing the effectiveness of your workout. So don't make the mistake of underestimating the importance of this part of the program. Even if for some reason you cannot complete all of the preparatory movements, be sure to do some of them each time you work out, right before you move on to the toning exercises.

Each particular exercise has a recommended number of repetitions, but if you feel your body is not loosening up sufficiently, then repeat the movements a few more times until you begin to feel a greater ease of movement in the joints and the rest of the body. There are many factors that determine how quickly you are able to warm up. The time it takes will depend on the time of day you choose to do your workout, how active you have been prior to starting and whether your mind is preoccupied with other matters. So be aware that on some days you will move through your warm-up more quickly and with greater ease than on others. Do take note of those

GEARING UP

occasions where you feel you've had an easier time of it. Perhaps you could adjust the time of your workout accordingly or place yourself in a similar environment. A good warm-up sets you up for an even better workout.

As you perform each warm-up movement, the more you can concentrate on the correct positioning, the more effective each repetition will become and the sooner your body will begin to loosen up.

Right, enough of that. Come on, let's get down to it. Remember, these movements are simple, fluid and smooth – the real work is yet to come!

LOW BACK RELEASE

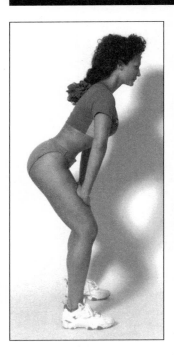

If your job involves a great deal of sitting during the day, you might want to practise this movement to give your back a bit of relief.

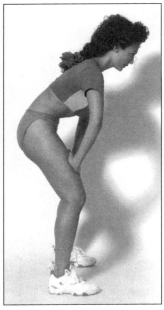

● Stand with feet a little wider than hip-width apart and place your hands on your thighs, well above the knees.

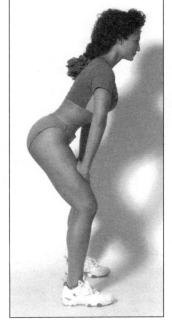

● Press your belly-button toward your low back and gently round your back, then come back to a flat back position. Round over again, then back to a flat back. Continue like this, running smoothly through the movements 16 times, each time making sure you flatten and then hollow out the low back as much as you can.

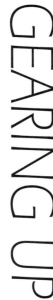

HIPS AROUND THE WORLD

- Start with feet shoulder-width apart, hands on hips.

- Here, you are going to roll the hips in a full circle. Press the hips first to the back, then to one side, and then lift your abdomen and press your pelvis underneath you to flatten the low back. Keep going, moving the hips through to the other side, to the back again, and continue in the same direction. Repeat 8 times in a fluid movement, then repeat in the opposite direction. Be sure to do the same number of repetitions in each direction.

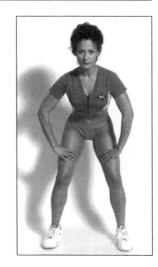

GEARING UP

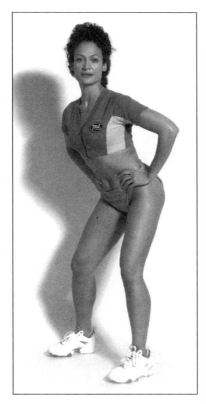

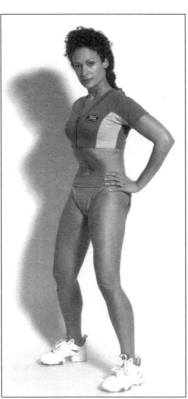

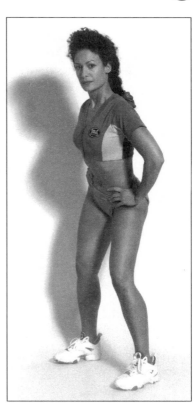

GEARING UP

THIGH STRETCHER

● Start with the back knee on the floor and the other leg in front with foot flat on the floor, hands on the floor at either side of the front foot. In this exercise you are going to move forward onto the front knee, so check the positioning of the front foot before you start. Be sure to place the front foot well beyond the knee so that as you move forward into position, your front knee ends up on top of the ankle, with the front leg at a 90-degree angle, and the back leg is nice and long, especially at the top of the thigh (hip joint). Keep your upper body lifted at all times.

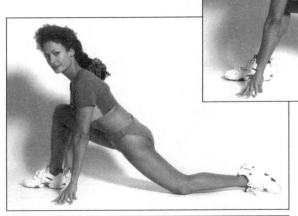

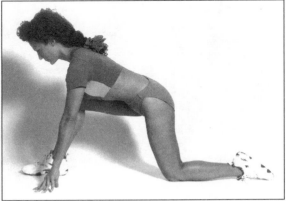

● Slowly bend the front knee and press forward, while maintaining the lift in your upper body. Hold for a count of 2, then slowly come back to the start position. Move into the stretch again and repeat the forward and backward movement 4 times. Each time you move forward, really feel that lift from your belly-button right through to the top of your head. On the last repetition, hold the thigh stretch for a count of 8.

● Switch legs, and repeat with the other leg in front.

ON THE RACK

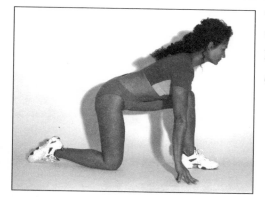

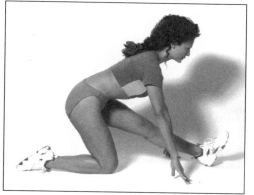

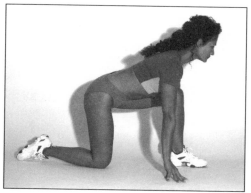

This is a great warm-up stretch for the hamstrings. Don't let the name put you off!

● Start with the back knee on the floor and the front leg bent, but this time make sure the knee is right on top of the ankle. Both hands are on the floor, at either side of the front leg. From here you are going to move your weight back, making sure that your weight does not rest directly on the kneecap of the supporting leg, but just below it.

● Straighten your front leg, raising the toes off the floor and lifting your belly-button, along with your upper body, up and over toward your extended leg. Take care *not to sit on your back leg*, as this will place pressure on the ligaments of the knee. Move forward to the starting position and then back to a fully straightened leg. Repeat 4 times and on the fourth repetition, hold in the extended position for a count of 8.

GEARING UP

● Be sure to have both hands on the floor, or your muscles will contract instead of loosening. If you are unable to bring both hands down as you move back, try to bring the hand on the same side as the extended leg down to the floor.

● Switch legs and repeat.

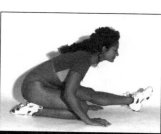

Sitting all the way back on the knee can damage the structures which hold the knee together.

GEARING UP

ANKLE CIRCLES

As we'll be doing a great deal of standing floor work later, we need to make sure the ankles are fully prepared for the work they will be undertaking.

- Stand with your hands on your hips and shift your weight onto one leg. Circle the other ankle outward and do 8–10 full rotations. Repeat, this time circling the ankle inward. Make the circles smooth and be sure to keep your weight off the circling ankle.

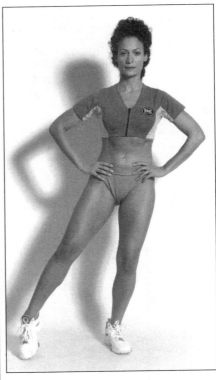

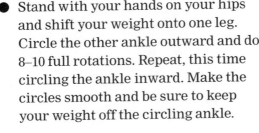

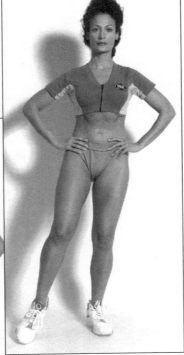

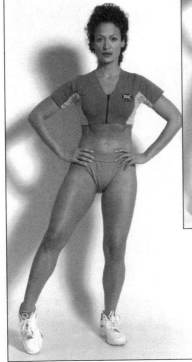

- Now repeat the whole sequence with the other ankle.

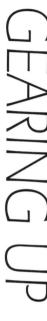

SIDE LUNGE STRETCH

- Stand with feet shoulder-width apart, hands on hips.

- Step the left leg out to the side and bend the knee, placing both hands well above the left knee and straightening the right leg. As you go down into the lunge, try to place your weight toward the hip area of the left leg so that you feel a stretch in the inner thigh of the right leg. To complete your next repetition, just straighten the left leg, then bend it again. Repeat 8–10 times and, on the last repetition, pull the toes up on the extended leg and hold the lunge position for a count of 8.

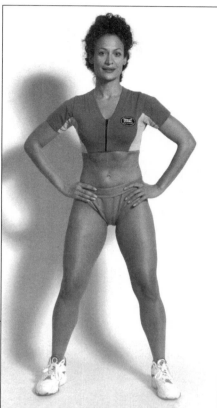

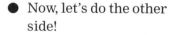

- Now, let's do the other side!

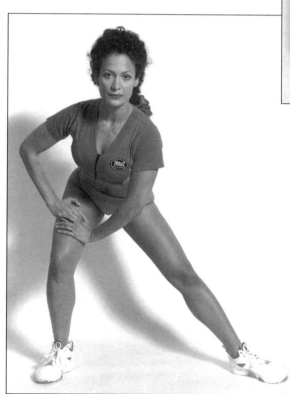

GEARING UP

2 7

GEARING UP

NECK RELIEF

You can also use this one to relieve any tension that may creep into the neck and shoulder area during the course of your day. If you've got children, a husband, wife or a demanding boss, then you'll have tension in this area. Sometimes when we're concentrating really hard on an exercise, or indeed any task, this tension tends to make us lift our shoulders. Be aware of this tendency and try to keep your shoulders down and relaxed at all times, not just when working out but also throughout the rest of the day. Come on, let's try and get rid of some of that tension.

● Stand with feet shoulder-width apart, hands on hips, shoulders back and down.

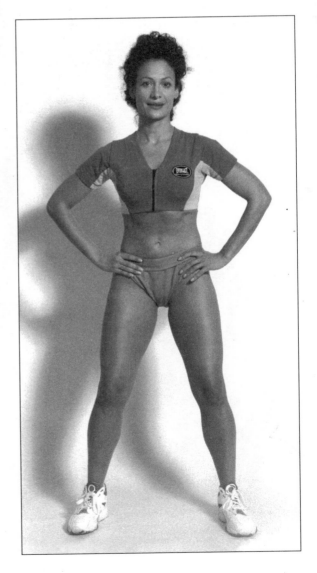

● Bring one arm up and place your hand on the opposite side of your head. Gently let your head fall to one side, applying a little pressure just above your ear to help the head lengthen away from the pressed-down shoulder. Hold for a count of 16. Now, still holding your head to one side, tilt your chin up slightly and hold for a further count of 16.

● If your neck is really tight, you may find it uncomfortable to hold for 16 counts. If this is the case, hold for 8 counts, take a short break and then hold for a further 8 counts.

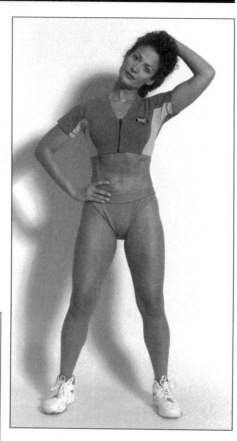

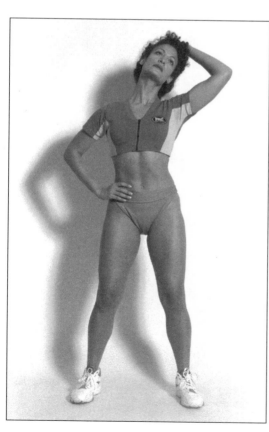

● Don't forget to repeat on the other side.

● Finish off by just letting your head rock, ear to shoulder, from one side to the other 8 times in a fluid, smooth fashion.

● If you still feel some tension in this area, repeat the exercise on both sides, giving yourself another 8–16 counts in each position.

GEARING UP

REACH AROUND

In this one, you need to think L O N G. Think of reaching from your waist, feeling your energy flow through your torso right up to your fingertips. Try to keep the shoulders down and away from your ears.

● Stand with feet shoulder-width apart, hands on hips. Take one arm and reach straight up. When you have stretched up as far as you can, start to reach over to the side in a smooth motion, coming forward from the waist slightly to move the stretch from your side into your back. Return to the start position and repeat to the other side.

● Alternate sides, doing 4–8 repetitions to each side, maintaining a smooth, seamless and circular quality in your movement. If you find that any part of this stretch hits an area that feels really tight, hold there for a little while.

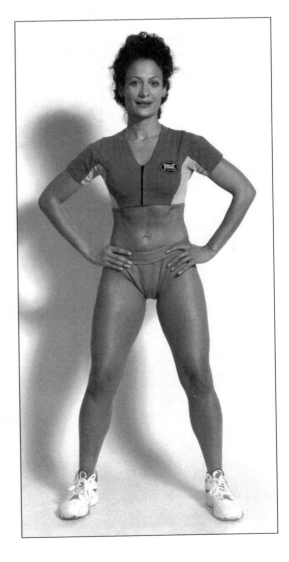

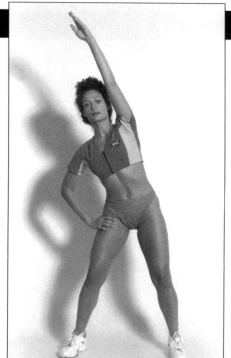

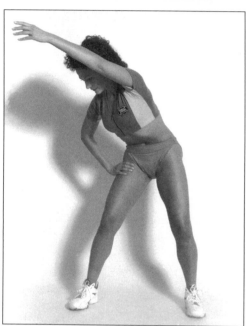

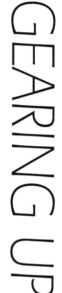

GEARING UP

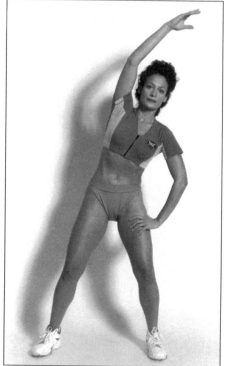

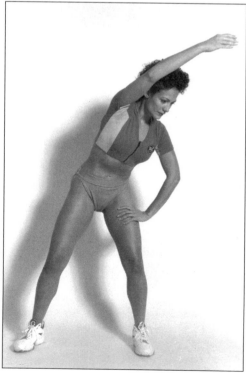

GEARING UP

QUAD ELONGATOR

● The front of the thighs are very rarely stretched completely during our everyday activities, so it's important to take time to lengthen them and warm them up. Position yourself carefully in this exercise, and you'll feel a stretch in the whole of the front of the thigh. Use the back of a chair, sofa or a wall for support.

● Hold onto your support with your right hand. The other hand remains free to hold the foot of the leg being stretched. Bend the left knee until you can grab hold of your foot, preferably the heel, while lifting your abdomen up and keeping your pelvis underneath you to avoid arching the back.

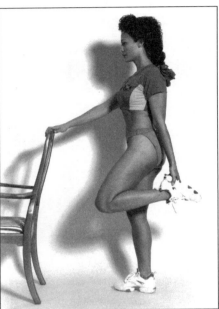

● Move the knee back *without arching your low back*. You should feel the top of your left thigh begin to stretch. When the knee is as far back as you can take it, bring the heel toward your buttocks just a little. Hold for a count of 10–20. Ahhhhh!

● You'll know if you are pressing the knee too far back, because the low back will start to arch and you'll feel tension in this area. In the correct position, you should feel the whole of the front of the thigh lengthen without any strain on the knee or low back.

● Are you ready to do the other leg?

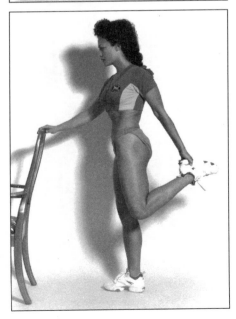

> **Are you feeling nice and warm? Come on, let's move on to the part of the program where we are going to make some real changes!**

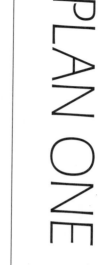

Plan One:
Lean Technique

Straight Squat

Power Legs

Easy Chair Extensions

Leg Works

High Hip Twister

Inner Thigh Roll

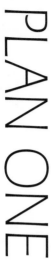

PLAN ONE

Have you warmed up? Ok, then it's time to familiarize yourself with the basics. Each exercise in this plan has been chosen to demonstrate the basic muscle function and help you find your proper positioning.

Try to think of each exercise as a controlled, continuous, fluid series of movements that you follow through, one after the other. To get the most out of each exercise, hold firmly and upright at the end of each repetition for 2–3 seconds, just long enough to really concentrate on your placement before you commence the next repetition. Then, as you return to the starting position, anticipate your move right into the next repetition. Although guidelines are given for repetitions, don't worry if you are unable to complete the suggested number at first. Gradually work up to the recommended amount. If you want to do more, then go ahead! Always be sure to do an equal number on each side. Once you feel confident with an exercise, you can aim to complete another set.

You want these exercises to hit your bottom line, so do make absolutely sure you acquire a good working knowledge of the correct positioning. To make continued progress it is essential that you feel a certain amount of confidence and are able to complete the recommended number of repetitions in strong, clean form before moving on to the next plan. Concentrate on keeping your abdomen lifted throughout each exercise to help maintain your balance. Remember to squeeze your buttocks – if you keep them loose, they will stay loose!

I want you to see and feel results in as short a time as possible. So, apply yourself to the basics, and you'll get so much more out of the increasingly challenging exercises later in the program. Watch those legs change shape.

Let's get started!

STRAIGHT SQUAT

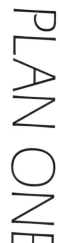

PLAN ONE

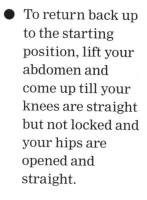

Take time to find your correct body positioning in this exercise. Use a mirror to check the alignment of your hips, knees and ankles. Your placement in this exercise is crucial to the execution of many of the exercises in this book, so it's worth spending some time on familiarizing yourself with it.

● Stand with feet shoulder-width apart and parallel, feet pointing straight ahead, hands on hips. Your weight is balanced from the arches of your feet, toward your heels, and your knees are aligned above your ankles.

● Keeping your chest upright and your knees directly over your ankles, extend your arms forward while pushing your buttocks backward and bending your knees as if you were about to sit back on a chair.

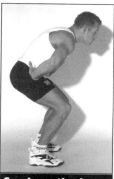

See how the knee takes a lot of abuse in the squat position if you allow your weight to go forward and knees to go past your ankles.

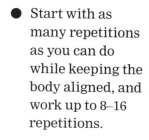

● To return back up to the starting position, lift your abdomen and come up till your knees are straight but not locked and your hips are opened and straight.

● Start with as many repetitions as you can do while keeping the body aligned, and work up to 8–16 repetitions.

TRAINER'S TIPS

▶ As you descend into the squat position, try not to let your knees go forward and avoid tucking your pelvis under – just sit back so that the knees remain above the ankles.

▶ When returning to the starting position, lift up from the abdomen and be sure to straighten the hips without locking the knees – try not to remain bent at the hips (top of the thighs).

POWER LEGS

PLAN ONE

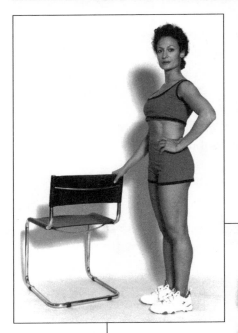

This lunge is fundamental to the functional floor work in this program, so be prepared to spend some time on finding your proper positioning. With practice, the properly aligned position will become second nature.

● Stand straight with feet together. Your left hand is on your hip and your right hand is resting on the back of a chair for support.

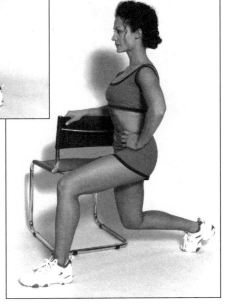

● Lift your abdomen and, keeping your upper body weight lifted and back, shift your weight onto your right leg and extend the left leg in front to go down into the lunge position, bending both knees and keeping your torso upright. The front knee should be aligned right over the ankle.

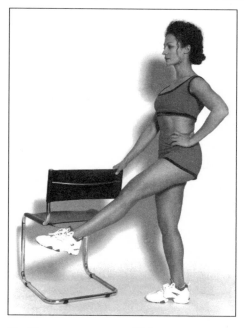

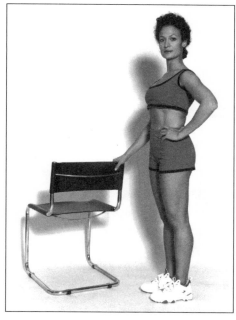

PLAN ONE

- To return to the starting position, lift your abdomen while squeezing your buttocks and push away from the floor. At this point, be sure to bring your upper body straight up and back to the starting position as you bring the feet together. Try not to lean forward.

- Do as many repetitions as you can, aiming for 8–16 complete, clean repetitions. By clean, I mean that as you descend into the lunge and as you push back up, make sure your body weight is not thrown forward or back. Instead, keep your upper body upright.

- Repeat on the other side. Be sure to do an equal number of repetitions on each side.

TRAINER'S TIPS

▶ During this exercise the abdomen stays lifted for balance and control.
▶ Make sure you squeeze the buttocks – if they remain loose, they will stay loose.
▶ Keep the front knee stable – try not to let it wobble either toward your body or away from you.

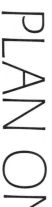

PLAN ONE

EASY CHAIR EXTENSIONS

This is an easy position in which to work the buttocks.

● Rest your forearms on the back of a chair. Press your shoulder blades down to keep your shoulders away from your ears, and keep your abdomen lifted to hold the pelvis in position. Bring one knee up in front.

● Now extend the leg down and to the back as if you were pushing an object away with your foot while keeping the rest of your body stationary, especially the hips.

● Bring the knee right up in front again to anticipate the next repetition. Imagine that someone is trying to push your leg toward your body while you are resisting and aiming to straighten the leg down and back.

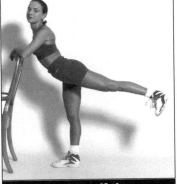

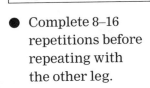

As you can see, if the abdomen is not lifted and you try to lift the leg too high, your back is greatly compromised and the exercise is much less effective.

TRAINER'S TIPS

► As you extend the leg, the more you are able to keep the rest of the body stationary, the more successful you'll be in targeting the buttock muscles.

► Although you are using the chair for support, take care not to allow your body to slump completely into the chair. Keep the body upright and ensure only the working leg moves.

● Complete 8–16 repetitions before repeating with the other leg.

LEG WORKS

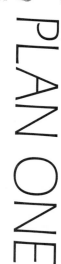

PLAN ONE

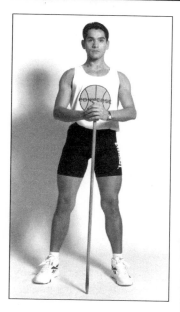

You'll need to use a broomstick or pole in this exercise.

● Stand and hold your broomstick or pole in front of you at a comfortable distance. Your elbows should not be too close to your body, yet your arms should not be extended to such an extent that your body position is thrown off centre because you're reaching too far.

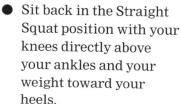

● Sit back in the Straight Squat position with your knees directly above your ankles and your weight toward your heels.

● Now, without letting your shoulders raise, lift up from the abdomen and squeeze your buttocks under you as you move the body straight up while lengthening one leg out to the side. The raised knee remains facing forward.

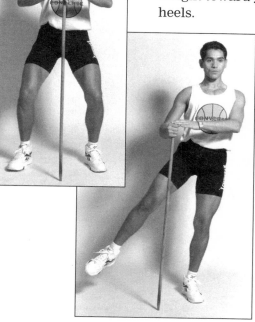

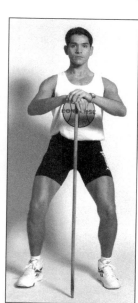

● Keep the movement controlled as you come back down into the squat position and then lift your upper body to raise and lengthen the opposite leg. Aim for 10–14 repetitions, alternating legs.

TRAINER'S TIP

▶ The body should remain lifted from the hips, fighting the forces of gravity. The supporting leg pushes into the ground and the working leg reaches out to the side. Really get into those outer thighs! The more you are able to keep the body upright and maintain the lift in your abdomen, the longer your range of movement will be, allowing you to lift the leg well out to the side, and the greater the work for the outer thigh muscles.

PLAN ONE

HIGH HIP TWISTER

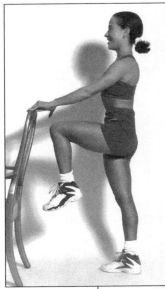

- Stand upright and rest your hands on the back of a chair. Shift your weight onto one leg and lift the other knee up in front.

- Using the raised knee, trace a quarter circle around and away from the centre of the body. As you bring the knee out to the side, try not to drop the leg or allow the hips to shift out of position.

- Bring the knee to the front again and repeat. Keep your buttocks tightly squeezed under at all times. If you bring your pelvis under you and lift your abdomen, this will ensure your hips are in the correct position.

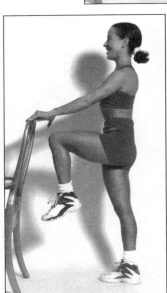

- Aim for 8–16 repetitions, then repeat with the other leg.

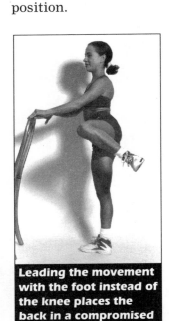

Leading the movement with the foot instead of the knee places the back in a compromised position and renders the exercise ineffective.

TRAINER'S TIP

▶ Think of opening the lifted leg away from the centre of your body, while keeping the rest of the body still. It's a very 'quiet' movement. Although the knee moves to the side, the movement comes from the hip and tightened buttocks.

INNER THIGH ROLL

Now, in this relatively comfortable position, we're going to do some work on the inner thighs and buttocks. Find yourself a ball – a beach ball or football – to use in this exercise.

- Sit on the floor with knees bent and feet flat on the floor. Place the ball between your knees, then lower your upper body to the floor, using your hands to support you and keeping your abdomen lifted. Once on the floor, you can relax the upper body into the floor. Squeeze the ball, pressing against it with your inner thighs, and try to maintain this contraction throughout the exercise.

- Once you have a good grip on the ball, tighten your buttocks and start curling your tailbone up toward the ceiling, rolling from the base of the spine. Keep tightening your buttocks and squeezing your inner thighs as you tilt the pelvis under on a slow count of 1…2…3…4.

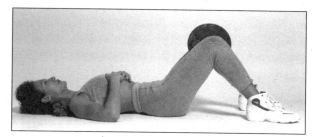

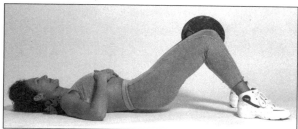

- Release the pelvic tilt just a little, but keep squeezing your inner thighs – in other words, don't let go of the ball. Again, tighten your buttocks and tilt the pelvis under on a slow count of 4.

- Aim to complete 4 repetitions of this sequence, maintaining the contraction in your inner thighs throughout.

Yes, you did it! You've completed your first workout and are on the way to acquiring beautiful, strong legs. Your muscles are now nice and warm which is a good time to increase your flexibility. So turn to page 81 for a series of stretches that will leave you on a high note as you wind down.

PLAN ONE

TRAINER'S TIP

▶ Note that my hands are resting on my ribcage to ensure that I am not pressing against the floor with them to assist in the pelvic tilt. Instead, I am tilting the pelvis by squeezing my buttocks and lifting my abdomen. Most of the back should remain on the floor.

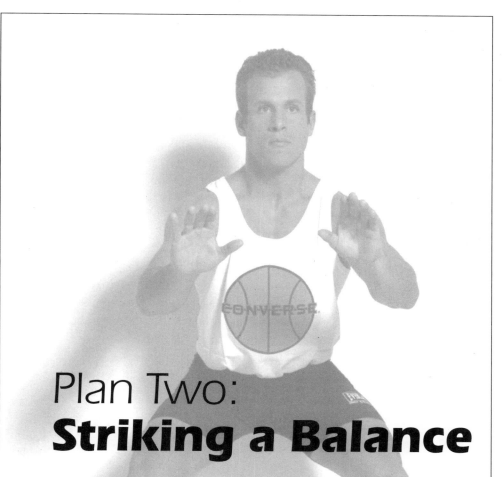

Plan Two:
Striking a Balance

Outer Thigh Eraser
Static Rotators
Low Hip Twister
Upright Extension
Pole Plié
Lateral Traveller
Complete Leg
Thigh Tamer

PLAN TWO

Is your body and mind in gear? Remember always to do the simple warm-up movements on pages 22–32 before you start your toning workout.

You have mastered Plan One, so your strength must be improving. Focus on those aspects of your training that are real for you. Are you finding it easier to hold a bent leg position? Can you sense the strength gains in your abdomen as well as your legs?

In this plan we're raising the stakes. Now that you're familiar with the basics, it's time to test your sense of balance and use it to your advantage in improving your posture and exercise technique.

We'll also start to introduce some travelling moves to add another dimension to your program so that you can really begin to complete each exercise in a dynamic way. At this stage, we are not yet looking to develop speed – that will come later, along with your strength gains. We're simply testing the water. What we are aiming to accomplish is to move dynamically through the exercises by lifting and contracting the muscles in unison. The movement sequences are a bit longer, and this will drive up the intensity level and provide your muscles with a stimulus that more closely resembles natural, everyday movements.

Remember, as you perform each exercise, the more you can concentrate on the correct positioning, the more effective each repetition will become and you'll be yet another step closer to the way you want to look and feel. So, stick in there.

Come on, let's go!

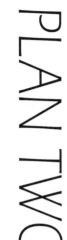

OUTER THIGH ERASER

Guess what we're going to chisel away at in this exercise!

- Lie on your side with knees slightly bent and one arm folded comfortably under your head. The other arm is in front of your body, with palm flat on the floor to assist your balance. Lift the top leg as high as you can, keeping the leg slightly bent and making sure the knee remains facing forward. Avoid pointing the knee upward as you lift the leg, since this will take the work away from the outer thigh and throw you off balance.

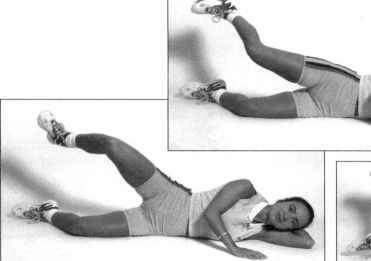

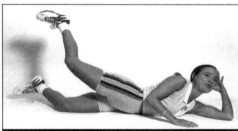

Oops! Look at the abdomen and back. They must remain lifted or the back will get compressed.

- Once you have lifted the leg to its full range, while holding your hips in place and not allowing the top hip to roll back, turn the leg out. When the leg reaches its full turn-out position, bring it to face forward again, then take it down to the floor. Go right into your next repetition. This sequence continues straight through for 8–16 repetitions.

- Be sure to complete the same number of repetitions on the other side.

TRAINER'S TIPS

▶ When lifting the leg or turning it out, if you lean just a little into the front hand on the floor, this will help prevent you from leaning back.

▶ If you tilt your pelvis underneath you as you turn the leg out, this will help you to hold the hips in place and also work the buttocks and the rotators (a small group of muscles located just under the gluteals).

PLAN TWO

PLAN TWO

STATIC ROTATORS

This exercise targets the rotators, a small group of muscles located under the gluteal muscles. The rotators work in tandem with the buttock muscles.

- Grab a ball and place it between your feet. Lie face down on the floor and rest your face on your hands. Squeezing the ball tightly with your feet, lift your heels up and bend your knees. Turn your knees out to the side just a little, keeping them on the floor, and squeeze the ankles and feet together. Hold for a count of 4.

- Open the knees a little more and squeeze the ball once again with the feet and ankles, holding for another count of 4. If you can turn your knees out a bit further without losing the ball, go for another count of 4.

- Take a break if you need to. But try to hold the legs for a count of 4 in at least three different angles of turn-out.

- Try to complete two full rounds, each time holding for 4 counts in the three positions.

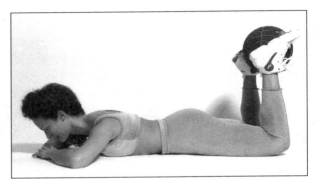

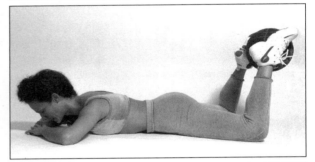

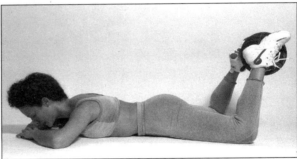

TRAINER'S TIPS

▶ You'll get the most out of this exercise if you continuously hold your abdomen in and up, away from the floor, to help keep your back down.

▶ Try not to get frustrated if the ball slips away from you. As your strength and control increases, it will become much easier to hold the ball in place and you'll feel a real sense of accomplishment.

LOW HIP TWISTER

This is similar to the High Hip Twister in Plan One, but here the leg is in a lower position. Use a broomstick or pole in this exercise for additional support. Remember, however, the lift in your abdomen is going to be your main source of support.

● Stand with feet apart and hold the broomstick or pole comfortably in front of you, aligned with the centre of your body. Shifting your weight onto one leg, lift the other knee in front.

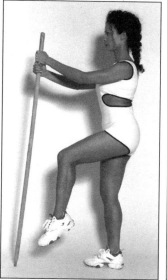 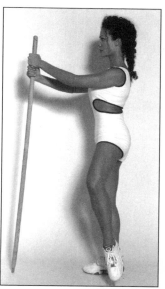 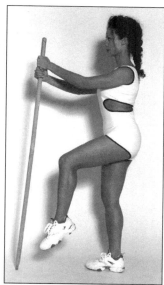

● Now, using the raised knee, trace a quarter circle around and away from the centre of your body and place the raised foot by the ankle of the standing leg. Your waist and buttocks remain stationary as the knee moves away from the body as much as possible, and your buttocks are squeezed tightly under you. Hold in this position until the hips feel square and the raised leg is turned out as far as it will go.

● Keeping your buttocks tightly tucked under, reverse the movement to return to the starting position so that the knee is once again lifted in front.

● Repeat as many times as you can properly, working up to 16–20 repetitions in correct form, then repeat on the other side.

TRAINER'S TIPS

▶ Aim to keep the shoulders back and down, using the lift in your abdomen to maintain an upright position.

▶ Really try to avoid moving the hips in this exercise. Keep them facing straight ahead.

▶ Remember, your broomstick is just an aid, so keep your weight pulled up and away from it instead of leaning all your weight onto it.

PLAN TWO

PLAN TWO

UPRIGHT EXTENSION

This is a great one for the buttocks and the hamstrings (back of the thighs).

● Stand with the broomstick or pole in front of you at a comfortable distance so that your shoulders are down and not straining to hold the broomstick in place.

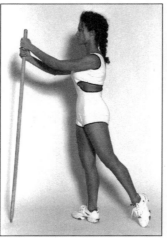 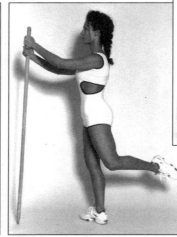

● Extend one leg to the back, tracing the floor with your foot so that your leg is straight behind you. Make sure the movement comes from the hip (top of the thigh), keeping it away from the low back, and avoid pushing the leg too far. At the correct position you will feel a strong contraction in the buttocks. This is your starting position. If you continue to push the leg back, there will come a point where your pelvis will shift into an arched position and you will feel it in your low back. If this happens, you have taken the leg too far.

● Now lift the heel toward your buttocks, making sure the knee does not come forward and that your pelvis remains upright as in the starting position. Bring the foot back down to tap the floor, pelvis still upright, and you're ready for your next repetition. Try 8–16 repetitions before moving to the other leg.

TRAINER'S TIPS

▶ To get the most out of this exercise, you must not allow your back to arch. If you feel a release in the contraction in your buttocks, then you are arching the back. Keeping your abdomen lifted will help you hold the proper position.

▶ If necessary, start from the beginning to reposition the toe correctly on the floor for the next repetition.

POLE PLIÉ

Here we can hit the inner thighs, outer thighs, hamstrings and buttocks. The trick is not to slump as you lower your body into the plié but to remain pulled up throughout. Use your broomstick or pole for added support.

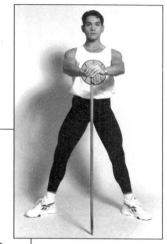

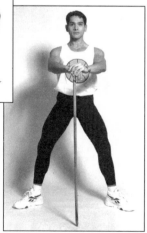

- Stand with feet shoulder-width apart and hold the broomstick or pole at a comfortable distance away from your body so that your arms are lengthened. Make sure the broomstick or pole is centred in front of your body. Turn your legs out, first from the hips, then followed by the knees, ankles and feet.

- Bend your knees, pressing them out toward the sides of the room, and go down into your plié, making sure you remain pulled up from the waist. Your bottom should remain under your hips throughout the whole of the movement. Press the knees right out to the sides and go down as far as you can, keeping your heels on the floor and making sure that your knees do not bend more than 90 degrees. If they bend further than this it will overload the work on the knees and hips, so just keep pressing your knees out to the sides and back.

- Come back up to the starting position and repeat. Try to complete 10–16 repetitions.

Note: Unlike in a squat, the hips do not move back but remain right underneath you, and as you bend the knees the legs press open and out toward the sides of the room. Once in the plié, you can tell if your turn-out is correct by looking over your knees – if you can see your toes sticking out in the same direction as the knees, then you are in the correct position.

PLAN TWO

TRAINER'S TIP

▶ Remember to go easy on the pole. Try not to hang onto it or use it to lift you up. The lift comes from your abdomen, not the pole.

4 9

PLAN TWO

LATERAL TRAVELLER

Here, we will be working the inner and outer thighs in a truly dynamic way.

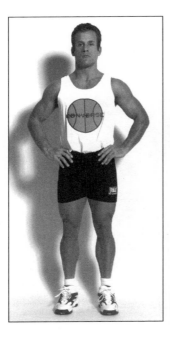
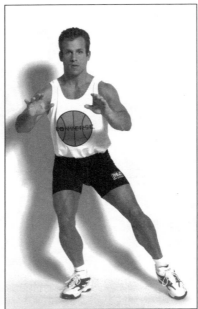
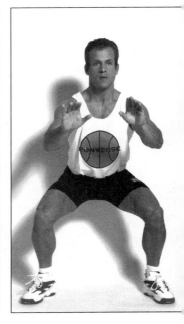

TRAINER'S TIP

▶ The width of your side-step will determine how deeply you bend the knees. We each have our own rhythm which affects how wide we step and how far we bend the knees. Try to deliberately alter your rhythm by either stepping wider or narrower than you would naturally.

● Stand straight with feet hip-width apart and hands on hips. You are going to bend the knees and prepare to shift your weight onto your left side. As you bend the knees, extend your right leg out to the side, raising your arms in front for balance. Then step out wide with the extended right leg and lower your body into a wide squat position so that your weight is now on both legs. Shift your weight onto your right side and keep moving in the same direction by bringing the left leg in to meet the right leg so that the feet are together and your body is up again.

● Now, begin to shift your weight onto your left side again while extending your right leg to keep travelling in the same direction. The movement is step to the side with legs wide, knees bend, trail leg comes in and body comes up. Get a rhythm going – side step, squat, trail leg in, side step, squat, trail leg in. Your body moves down, up, down, up. Be sure to really bend the knees well.

PLAN TWO

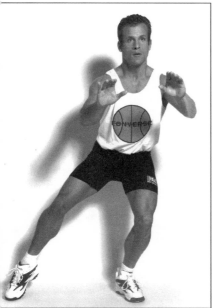

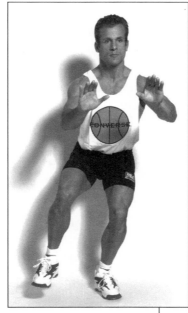

● Move in the same
direction for 8–16
counts, depending on
how much room you
have to travel in, then
repeat to the other side.

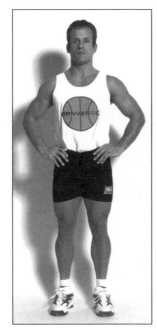

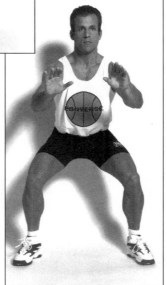

5 1

PLAN TWO

COMPLETE LEG

This is one of my favourites because it hits all the leg muscles, especially the buttocks. You will need a box or step for this exercise, or you can use the first step of the stairs in your home. Make sure the box is stable and capable of supporting your body weight. It should be at a height that ensures your knee does not bend beyond 90 degrees when you step up onto it.

● Stand in front of the box and place your right foot on top and in the centre of the box.

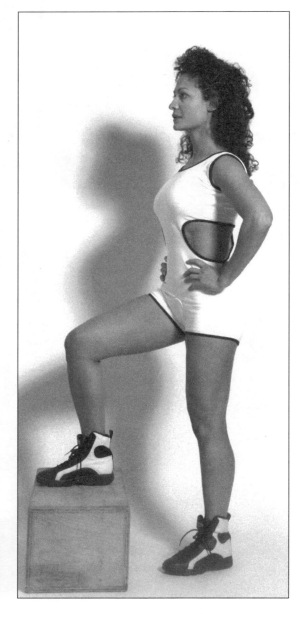

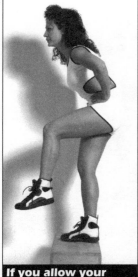

If you allow your body to collapse forward, as shown here, you will lose your balance.

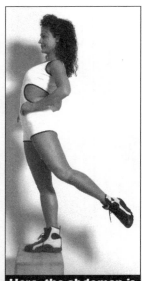

Here, the abdomen is released and the leg is forcefully thrown back which can hurt your back.

PLAN TWO

● Lift your abdomen and bring the left leg up in front in a knee lift, making sure your upper body moves straight up. Squeezing your buttocks tightly, extend the raised leg back in a controlled fashion, and really try to lengthen the leg. Imagine you are pressing an object away with your foot. Keep the hips square throughout and be sure to let the movement come from the tightening of your buttocks, rather than letting your abdomen sink and allowing the back to arch.

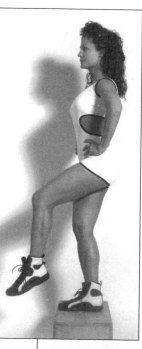

● Step back down to the floor with the raised left leg, making sure you bend the knee as you step down. Your right foot remains on the box so that you are ready to start your next repetition on the same leg.

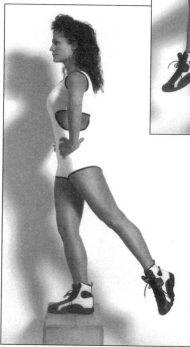

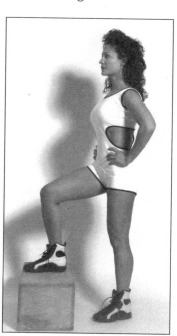

● Complete 8–16 repetitions on one leg, then repeat with the other leg. Of course, if you want to do more repetitions, that's great, as long as you remember to maintain a tall, lifted torso.

TRAINER'S TIPS

▶ As you extend the leg back, make sure your abdomen is lifted to help hold your pelvis in place. Really concentrate on ensuring this movement originates from the front of the hip (top of thigh).

▶ Keep your eyes focused upward and avoid looking down. Let this upward focus be reflected in your body. Keep your torso lifted and tall, and just step lightly on the foot as it comes back down to the floor.

5 3

THIGH TAMER

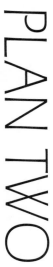

PLAN TWO

This exercise really targets the buttocks, but the bending of the knee also brings the added benefit of working the hamstrings. You will need to use some form of support, so find a piece of furniture such as a bureau or chair that is around chest height.

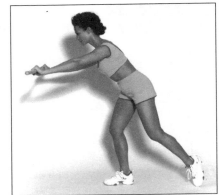

● Place your hands on the bureau or chair and position yourself so that your body is bent forward with your low back flat. Bend your knees slightly and move one leg back, keeping the knee bent and the big toe touching the floor. This is your starting position.

● Keeping your body bent forward and without arching your back, straighten the back leg. Concentrate on lengthening the leg until it is fully extended. Eventually, the leg will come up off the floor. Lifting your abdomen will allow you to open your leg fully at the hip, enabling you to really tighten your buttocks.

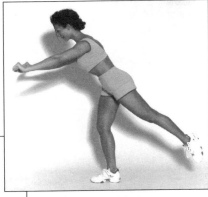

TRAINER'S TIPS

▶ Keeping your body bent forward and your low back flat during all your repetitions places the active leg in an advantageous position to work against gravity.

▶ The emphasis in this movement is on lengthening the leg so that you spend the maximum amount of time working against the pull of gravity. As you return to the starting position, anticipate your move right into the next repetition as soon as your toe touches the floor.

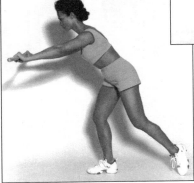

● Release and return to the starting position. The moment your toe touches the floor move straight into the next repetition. Do 8–16 repetitions, then repeat on the other leg.

Another workout completed and your legs are getting stronger and more shapely. Don't forget to turn to page 81 to do your stretches and gently wind down.

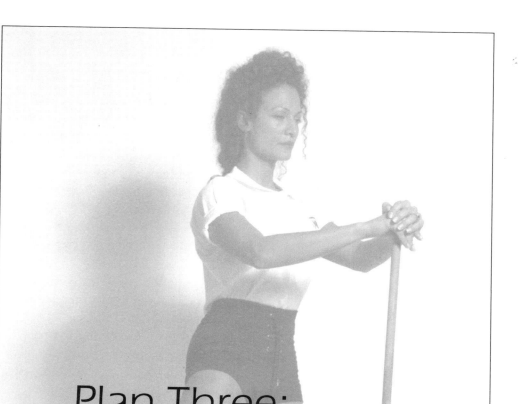

Plan Three:
Changing Tactics

Lateral Leg Lifter
Free Lunge
Pendulum Lunge
Three Point Lunge
Standing Scissors
Butt Rotator
Gravity Press
Butt Blaster

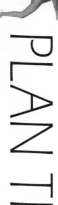

PLAN THREE

So, you're heading into Plan Three. Great! Are you feeling warm and ready to work those leg muscles? If some of your joints still feel a little stiff, then repeat the warm-up movements for those particular areas.

You have conquered Plans One and Two and, by now, you should have the confidence and ability to use your abdomen for support, allowing you to really concentrate on the specific muscle action in each exercise and increase the intensity and efficiency of your workout. Aligning your shoulders, hips, knees and ankles is now becoming second nature and you should be carrying this acquired skill over into your daily standing posture.

In this plan, you'll find some interesting variations on traditional exercises performed in a horizontal lying position as well as some longer sequences of unsupported standing work to help you to cultivate further your sense of balance. Exercises like the Free Lunge and Lateral Leg Lift, once mastered, will really strengthen and tighten the buttocks, front and back thighs, inner and outer thighs. With the exception of the Three Point Lunge and the Pendulum Lunge, you will no longer be using external support in your standing floor work. This creates an extra challenge, as you will have to use your improved sense of balance to support your weight on one side of the body while maintaining proper alignment. The Three Point Lunge and Pendulum Lunge, however, are more complex series of movements and so you'll still need some additional support.

We'll also be doing some more specific rotation exercises and, for good measure, I've added a Butt Blaster exercise that incorporates the use of a resistance band. Remember, if you do not have a resistance band this exercise can still be performed successfully without it – just follow the instructions for positioning and go through the same motions without the band.

You now have the necessary skills for balance that you acquired in Plan Two. What you want to do now is to enhance your control of it. You *can* do it. I know you can. So, let's move on to the more demanding series of exercises that I have planned for you here. You're well on your way!

LATERAL LEG LIFTER

In this exercise we are targeting the outer thigh muscles in addition to training our sense of balance.

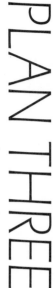

PLAN THREE

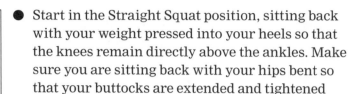

- Start in the Straight Squat position, sitting back with your weight pressed into your heels so that the knees remain directly above the ankles. Make sure you are sitting back with your hips bent so that your buttocks are extended and tightened rather than having your pelvis tucked under.

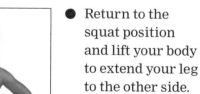

- Squeeze your buttocks and use your abdomen to lift your body straight up while lengthening one leg out to the side. The leg will ultimately come off the floor, but you should focus on lengthening rather than lifting the leg so that you aim to keep your hips level. Resist the temptation to allow one side of the hip to raise too high as the leg moves to the side.

- Return to the squat position and lift your body to extend your leg to the other side.

- Aim for 10–18 repetitions on alternate legs.

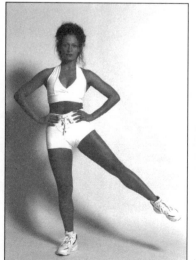

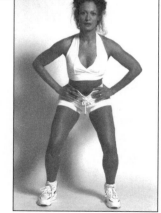

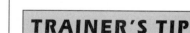

TRAINER'S TIP

▶ The more you lift your body straight up rather than allowing it to lean to one side, the more you will isolate the outer thigh muscles. This has the added benefit of training your abdomen to hold you upright.

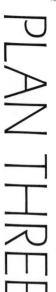

PLAN THREE

FREE LUNGE

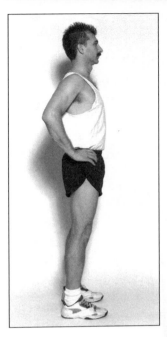

In this Free Lunge we hit just about all the leg muscles. The added bonus is that this is also a good exercise to develop your sense of balance. When descending into your lunge, your upper body remains centred directly above both legs.

● Stand with hands on your hips and lift your abdomen, feeling the energy flow from your feet right up through the top of your head.

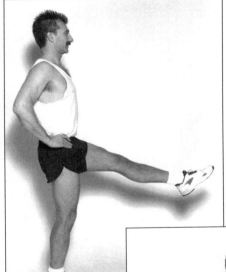

● Now lift your abdomen further and extend one leg, really lengthening the leg to go forward and down into the lunge position where the front knee is bent no more than 90 degrees.

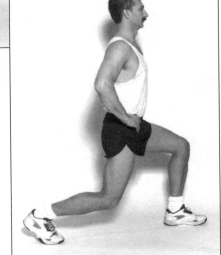

PLAN THREE

● Push up with that same leg to come back to the starting position, then prepare to lunge forward with the other leg.

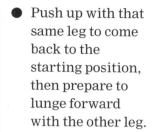

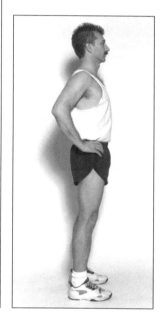

● For the first week or so that you practise this exercise, alternate legs, completing 8–16 repetitions. Once you get the hang of it, try doing 8–16 repetitions straight through on one leg before repeating with the other leg.

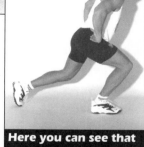

Here you can see that the weight is too far forward. This greatly increases the pressure in the front of the knee, putting most of the strain on the front thigh and taking away the concentration on the buttocks.

TRAINER'S TIPS

► When moving forward into the lunge or returning to the centre, make sure you keep your upper body directly on top of your centre point of balance between both legs.

► Really make an effort to avoid bending the upper body too far forward. Overloading the weight over the knee in this fashion will cause discomfort and, if a great deal of pressure is applied, could lead to injury.

PENDULUM LUNGE

PLAN THREE

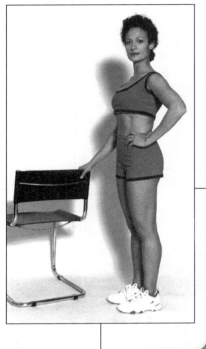

Here, we are using all the key leg muscles – the buttocks, inner and outer thighs and hamstrings.

● Stand upright and rest your right hand on the back of a chair for support. Your left hand is on your hip.

● Lift your abdomen and extend the left leg forward. Keep lengthening the leg and go into a full lunge position, making sure that the front knee bends no further than 90 degrees. Your upper body remains upright.

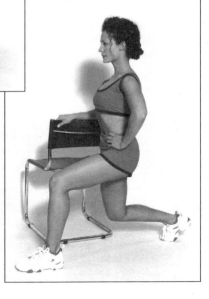

TRAINER'S TIPS

▶ Really pulling up with your abdomen will ensure that your body remains upright and also reduces the possibility of placing any undue stress on your low back.
▶ Keep your torso evenly balanced between both legs to ensure that your body does not collapse forward as you lunge to the front or that your body weight does not lean forward as you push up from the back lunge.
▶ Be sure to take the leg through its full range of motion when lunging to the back.

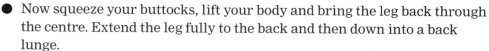

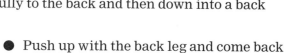

- Now squeeze your buttocks, lift your body and bring the leg back through the centre. Extend the leg fully to the back and then down into a back lunge.

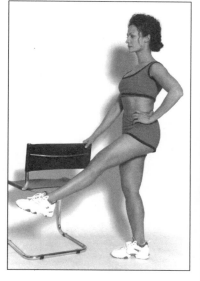

- Push up with the back leg and come back through the upright position ready to go straight down into your next forward lunge. Continue like this and complete your repetitions on this side before turning around and repeating with the other leg.

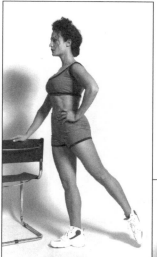

PLAN THREE

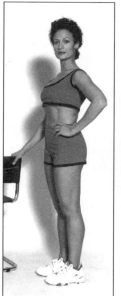

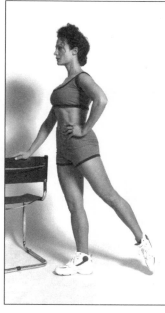

- Since you are using the same leg for some time, you may not be able to complete many repetitions at first, so aim for 6–8 repetitions. As you get stronger, you can increase the number as long as your body remains upright throughout the full movement. Within six weeks you could be up to 16 strong, clean repetitions.

61

THREE POINT LUNGE

PLAN THREE

In this exercise we get maximum benefits from all the leg muscles working together. Use a broomstick or pole for support.

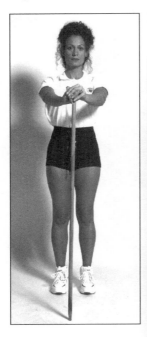

- Stand with the broomstick or pole out in front and aligned with the centre of your body.

- Lift your abdomen and extend one leg straight out in front and lower your body into a forward lunge, keeping the movement controlled and maintaining the lift in your upper body.

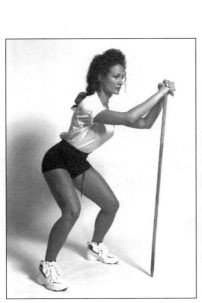

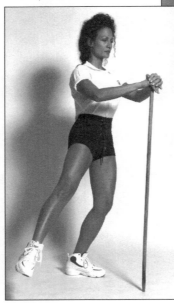

- Push yourself back up, with your body lifted straight up, then lengthen the same leg out to the side and smoothly lower into a squat position.

PLAN THREE

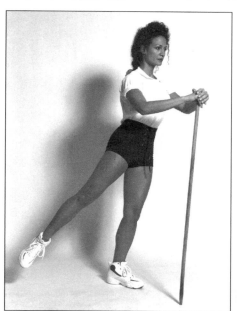

● Push the same leg away from floor and extend the leg to the back to descend with control into a back lunge.

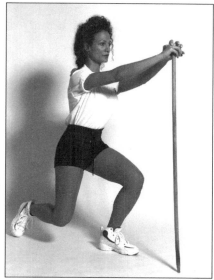

● Push away from the floor, aiming your body straight up and bring the leg to the centre in the starting position.

● Repeat the whole sequence with the other leg, aiming to complete 4 repetitions of the entire sequence on each side. Try to go straight through to each position and avoid holding onto the pole for dear life.

● If you want a real challenge, then try this sequence once on each side without the broomstick or pole so that you rely totally on your legs and abdomen for support.

TRAINER'S TIP

▶ The best way to develop your sense of control in this exercise is to accent the lifting part of each sequence and spend less time in the downward phase, so that you are actively resisting the attempts of gravity to pull you down. You are not going to allow any part of your body to droop without a real fight.

6 3

PLAN THREE

STANDING SCISSORS

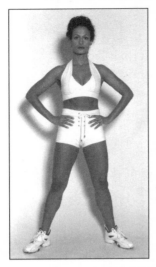

This one sculpts the inner thigh muscles. When nice and firm, these muscles can give a very attractive shape to the overall legs.

● Stand with legs apart and straight, without locking your knees. Allow your legs to turn out naturally from the hips a little, then follow with the knees and ankles so that they are all lined up.

● Now bend your knees into a plié position, then use the muscles of the legs and abdomen to lift your body straight up. As you lift up, place your full weight onto one leg and draw the other leg toward and slightly in front of the supporting leg in a scissor-like motion by squeezing the inner thigh muscles together.

● Return to bent knees and repeat to the other side. Continue with alternate legs, –16 repetitions on alternate legs. And you thought only dancers could have sculpted inner thighs!

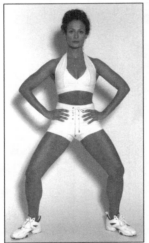

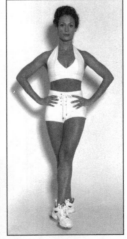

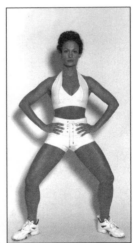

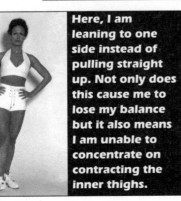

Here, I am leaning to one side instead of pulling straight up. Not only does this cause me to lose my balance but it also means I am unable to concentrate on contracting the inner thighs.

TRAINER'S TIPS

▶ Make sure you keep your hips directly underneath you rather than letting them move back as you bend the knees.

▶ Really concentrate on squeezing the inner thighs together to get the most out of this exercise.

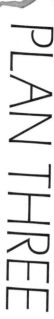

PLAN THREE

BUTT ROTATOR

For this exercise, you'll need a step or some form of box for support, about 12–16 inches (30–40 cm) high.

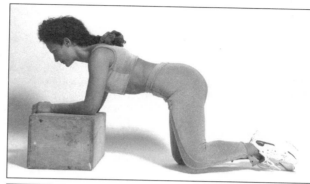

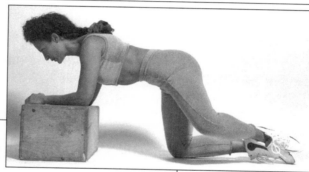

- Kneel in front of the box, with knees under hips and forearms relaxed on top of the box. Your back is extremely flat, from the top of your neck to your tailbone. Lift your left foot slightly off the floor and place your heels together. Your right knee remains on the floor to support your weight. The left knee is just off the floor and pointing down.

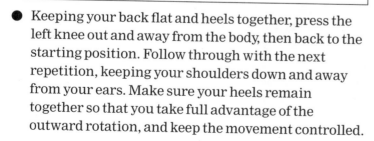

- Keeping your back flat and heels together, press the left knee out and away from the body, then back to the starting position. Follow through with the next repetition, keeping your shoulders down and away from your ears. Make sure your heels remain together so that you take full advantage of the outward rotation, and keep the movement controlled.

- Aim to complete 8–16 repetitions, then repeat on the other side.

TRAINER'S TIPS

▶ You need to maintain a flat back for the duration of the exercise. Keeping your abdomen lifted will help to hold your back in place. As the leg rotates out to the side, be sure to keep your low back very still instead of letting it move with the working leg.

▶ Should you find yourself leaning over into the supporting leg, place more weight onto the forearm on the same side as the working knee. This will allow you to distribute your weight more evenly on your three support points – both arms and the supporting knee.

PLAN THREE

GRAVITY PRESS

Follow the instructions closely in this exercise and you'll really feel it in your buttocks.

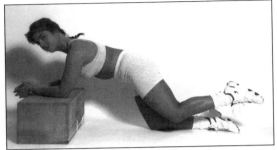

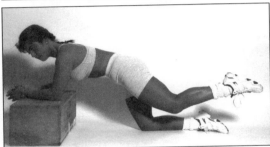

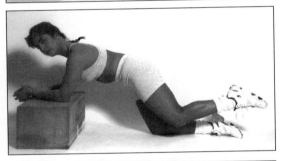

● Still kneeling in front of the box with your forearms resting on the box, keep one leg bent under you to act as a stabilizer and have the other leg slightly lifted off the floor with the knee still bent. This is your starting position.

● Lift your abdomen and press the raised leg back, letting the movement come from the front of the top of the thigh to open up the hip. Keep the knee relaxed and the movement controlled. Bring the knee down to the starting position, just off the floor, and work straight through for 8–16 repetitions. The objective is to extend the leg from the front of the top of the thigh on the working leg instead of letting the movement come from the low back.

● Completed your repetitions? Well, let's get ready to work the other side.

TRAINER'S TIPS

▶ It is important to keep the abdomen lifted tightly to keep the back as flat as possible and avoid placing stress on the low back.

▶ At first, you many find it difficult to keep the leg off the floor for the duration of your repetitions. If this is the case, then bring the leg all the way down for a short break. Bear in mind, though, to make this exercise a real winner, the ultimate aim is to keep the knee away from the floor for the full extent of your repetitions.

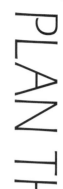

BUTT BLASTER

In this position you can really get into those buttock muscles and use the pull of gravity to your advantage. This exercise can be done with or without the resistance band or tubing.

- If you are using a resistance band or tubing, tie one end round the end of your foot and the other end to the leg of a sturdy chair. Now rest your weight on your forearms and knees. The leg you are going be working should be extended back slightly.

- Without lifting the leg, squeeze your buttock muscles on that side. Once you have tightened that side of the buttocks, follow through by lifting the leg. Your torso has nothing underneath to support it, so guess what you are going to use for support . . . ? Yes, that's right, the abdomen. Your abdomen must remain lifted throughout, otherwise your back will sink and this will place a great deal of stress on the spinal column.

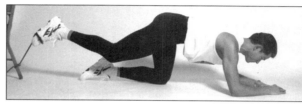
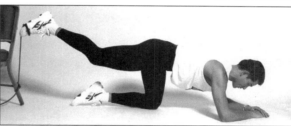
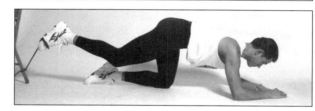

- Bring the leg down, but try to keep the knee off the floor. Do 8–16 repetitions, making sure you begin each repetition by squeezing the buttocks before you lift the leg. Remember to lift your abdomen each time you lift the leg.

- Repeat with the other leg. Be sure to do the same number of repetitions with each leg.

> **Great work! Now turn to page 81 to do your stretches and gently wind down.**

TRAINER'S TIP

▶ Your full range of motion for the leg in this position will be determined by how far you can lift the leg without arching your back or losing the support of your abdomen. Try to keep your back flat and maintain that position throughout each of your leg lifts.

PLAN THREE

Plan Four:
Right on Target

Travel Lunge
Plié to Lunge
Squat Jump
Frogs Legs
Bun Jump
All Fours Butt Lift
Rear Reconstructor
Butt Kicker

PLAN FOUR

Have you warmed up? Don't forget to repeat some of the warm-up movements if you feel you are not fully prepared.

OK, you have an improved sense of balance, and your legs and buttocks are getting tighter and firmer. So let's have some fun. In this plan I've added a spring to some of the exercises. I use the word 'spring' rather than 'jump' because the objective here, as in the rest of the program, is to complete the exercises in as controlled and safe a manner as possible. Whenever you add a spring, really concentrate on lifting with your whole body. Release the hip and knee joints on landing so that as you land *softly* the muscles do the work and you do not harm the joints by locking them. It's also important to maintain your correct alignment – shoulders over hips, hips over knees, knees over ankles – again to protect these joints.

One way of testing whether you are executing your spring correctly is to listen carefully as you land. If you are maintaining your body in an uplifted position and bending your knees well on landing, you should hear very little noise. On the other hand, if you're tired or just not ready for this challenge, you will hear a thud on landing, and the odds are your knees will not be above your ankles. If this is the case, review your technique and come back to that particular exercise at a later time. Once you are ready, however, the addition of these more powerful movements will further challenge your range of motion and change the speed at which you contract the muscles, helping you develop a more sculpted look. You'll both feel and see a real sense of power and strength in your legs.

Here, we also introduce several long sequences of movement, along with two very demanding travelling sequences. Once mastered, these will give you superior control of your body – not to mention tight legs.

Once you are proficient in each of the four plans, your sense of balance, your posture, your muscular strength and endurance and the shape of your legs and buttocks will all be greatly improved. You can then mix and match your favourite exercises from any of the plans. Just take care not to overwork any particular muscle group and be sure to include lots of variety. In chapter 4, The Bottom Line Break, you'll also find a number of variations to keep you progressing.

Let's get ready to go! Have fun.

TRAVEL LUNGE

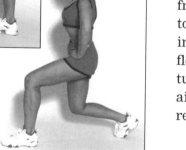

This is a challenging exercise which affects all the leg muscles, but pay careful attention to your correct alignment, especially the knees.

● Stand with feet together, hands on hips.

● Extend the left leg forward with control and go down into a forward lunge. Make sure the front knee bends no further than 90 degrees.

● Lift your body straight up, bringing the right leg in so that the legs are together. Now, extend the right leg forward and go down into a forward lunge. Lift the body straight up again, bringing the legs together.

● Continue to alternate legs so that you travel forward, moving across the floor in a controlled but fluid fashion. Make sure the front knee remains directly on top of the ankle as you descend into each lunge. Go across the floor as far as you can, then turn round and travel back, aiming to complete at least 16 repetitions.

Note: It is important to maintain the lift in your abdomen and keep your upper body aligned over the pelvis to avoid leaning forward and overstressing the joints, especially the knees. Allowing your upper body to lean forward will mean that most of the downward force in the exercise will be felt in the thigh of the front leg and therefore minimize the toning effect to the buttocks – which is not what you want. So, aim to keep your upper body centred, with your weight equally distributed between both legs, and remember to lift the body straight up between lunges.

PLAN FOUR

7 1

PLAN FOUR

PLIÉ TO LUNGE

Here we combine two major leg movements to create an exercise that will hit all your leg muscles. Note that the heel is lifted to allow you to adjust your position from forward to side. To check your alignment, look over your knees as you bend into the plié. Your feet should be facing the same direction as your knees.

● Stand with hands on hips and turn your legs out from the hips (top of the thighs). The knees follow suit, and the ankles and feet point in the same direction. It's always better to be a bit conservative and not attempt to turn the legs out further than your hips allow, otherwise the knees will be left in a vulnerable position.

● Bend your knees, pressing the legs open and aiming them to the sides of the room as you go down into a plié. Go down on counts 1…2, and come up 3…4. Repeat this cycle 4 times.

● Now, go down into your plié again and lift one heel. As you lift the heel, the hip, knee, ankle and foot on that side all turn at the same time so that you are now facing the side in a lunge position. Your upper body is lifted so that your weight is centred between both legs as you descend into your

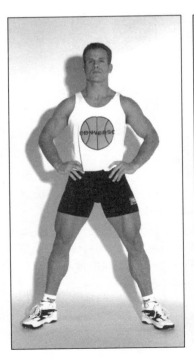
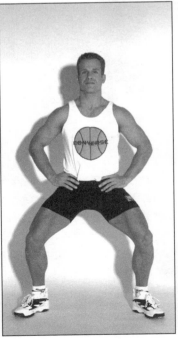
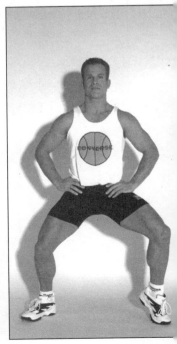

lunge. Go down 1…2, come up 3…4. Repeat this cycle 4 times.

● Come back to the centre and you are now ready to repeat the whole sequence, starting with your 4 pliés and then lifting the other heel and lunging to the opposite side. Aim to do 4 complete cycles, alternating sides.

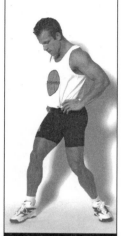

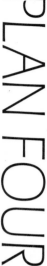

TRAINER'S TIPS

▶ Once you get into the rhythm of this one, try to execute the transition from the plié position to the lunge position in a smooth, seamless fashion. Keep your upper body lifted from your middle, not from your shoulders. Focus your mind on long and lifted.

▶ Look at the incorrect photograph and see the adverse effect on the knee joint if you do not lift the heel and have your joints lined up.

▶ Keep your head up. If you allow your head to drop forward, you'll find it difficult to line up the rest of the body.

As you can see, the knee is twisted and the foot and ankle are not in line with each other. Ouch!

PLAN FOUR

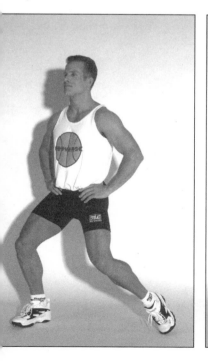

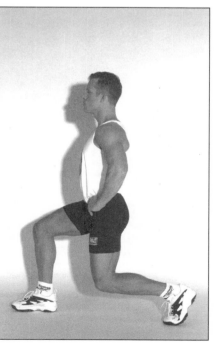

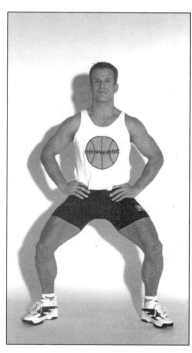

PLAN FOUR

SQUAT JUMP

This is an adaptation of the Straight Squat position. Here we are going to add a spring off the floor to help you develop a more explosive quality in your strength. This type of movement has the added benefit of increasing bone density. You don't have to jump very high, just enough to be able to straighten your legs fully and point your toes.

- Start by sitting back in your Straight Squat position.

- Lift your abdomen and spring right up off the floor, straightening the legs and pointing the toes.

- As you land, move through the feet, landing toe, ball, heel and then into bent knees and back into your basic squat position.

- As this is quite an intense movement, start off with just 6–8 repetitions. Don't forget to lift your abdomen as you spring up, and be sure to land smoothly by bending the knees.

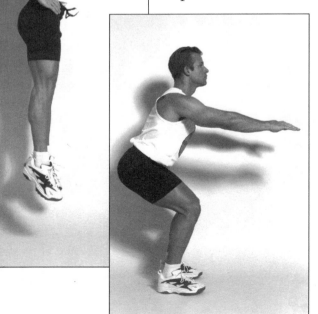

TRAINER'S TIP

▶ As kids we were always jumping up and down, so try to put yourself in a playful frame of mind as you do this exercise. It's just that now we know how to land correctly into those legs, we can utilize the springing action to strengthen and tone the buttocks and legs.

FROGS LEGS

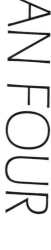

This position may look simple, but if you follow the instructions exactly, you'll feel a strong contraction in the buttocks, inner thighs and front of the thighs. Use your broomstick or pole for added support.

● Stand straight with heels together and legs turned out naturally. Try not to force too much of a turn-out as this will compromise your knees. Have your broomstick or pole in front of you, with your hands placed loosely on it.

● Pressing your heels down into the floor, bend your knees, opening them toward the sides of the room. Your buttocks remain directly underneath you. Continue to bend and open the knees until you feel your heels can no longer remain on the floor.

● Once you hit your lowest position, tighten your buttocks and keep them right underneath you as you lift your abdomen and start to straighten your legs, drawing the inner thighs together until the legs are completely straightened.

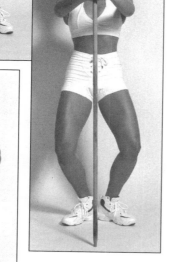

● Go right down into your next repetition, drawing the legs together really tightly as you come up again. Let's aim for 8–16 repetitions.

TRAINER'S TIPS

▶ Concentrate on keeping your buttocks directly underneath you. If the buttocks roll back, you will lose the contraction in this area and your buttocks will remain loose – which is not what you want!

▶ You'll know if you're doing this correctly because when the legs are completely straight you should feel the contraction in your buttocks, inner thighs and front of the thighs.

PLAN FOUR

BUN JUMP

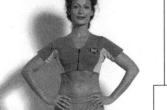

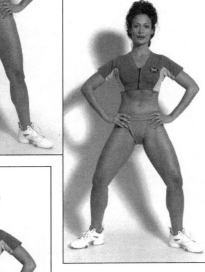

Here we are going to 'ignite' all the major leg muscles!

● Stand upright with legs apart, knees relaxed, feet turned out slightly and hands on hips.

● Bend your knees into a plié and use the impetus from this bending action to spring up just off the floor until the legs are fully straightened. *Make sure you bend the knees as you land.* Once you've landed, go down into your plié, ready to go right up into the next jump.

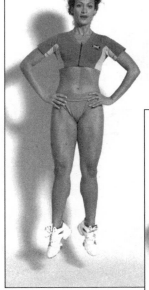

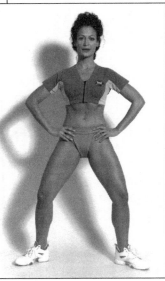

● Start with just 4–6 jumps and increase the number as you become stronger.

TRAINER'S TIPS

▶ Make sure you keep your body upright at all times. Avoid leaning forward as you jump or land, since this will throw you off balance.

▶ Be sure always to bend the knees as you land. Landing on straight legs would place a great deal of pressure on your low back and knees. Bending the knees helps protect the knees and low back in much the same way as shock absorbers in a car. It also ensures an extended contraction in the buttocks.

ALL FOURS BUTT LIFT

PLAN FOUR

This one is similar to the Butt Rotator in Plan Three but without the box for support. In this all fours position, it's extremely important to fully utilize the strength in your abdomen to keep your stomach pulled in and up and your low back flat. When lifting your leg in this position, the tendency is to allow the low back to curve and drop down toward the floor, placing a great deal of pressure on the base of the spine. But now that you've arrived at Plan Four you are well practised in using your abdomen for support and realize how important it is to maintain a stable, flat back.

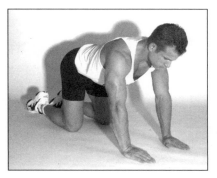

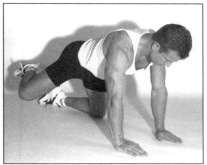

- Position yourself on your hands and knees on the floor, with knees about hip-width apart.

- Place your heels together and turn one knee away from the centre of your body so that the leg moves directly away from the supporting leg. Keep turning the knee out and the leg will eventually come off the floor.

- Bring the leg down to the starting position, then turn the knee out again to go straight into your next repetition.

- Aim for 8–16 repetitions, maintaining your flat back position throughout. Keep your shoulders down and try to keep your head lifted, not hanging down.

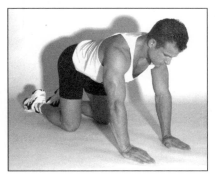

- Repeat with the other leg. Remember to do the same number of repetitions on each leg.

TRAINER'S TIP

▶ When lifting the leg from an all fours position, your weight naturally shifts to the opposite side of the body into the supporting leg. To balance this and avoid placing too much pressure on the supporting knee, try putting more weight on the arm on that side to distribute your weight more evenly between your support points.

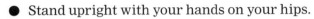

REAR RECONSTRUCTOR

PLAN FOUR

This exercise is a combination of the Travel Lunge and the Thigh Tamer so, done properly, it can be quite intense and can really improve your sense of balance.

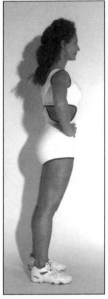

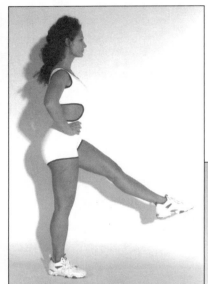

● Stand upright with your hands on your hips.

● Extend one leg forward, with the leg very straight to pull the thigh nice and tight.

● Move down into a forward lunge position, lowering the body straight down.

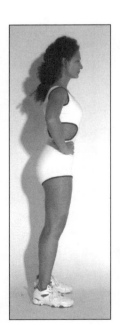

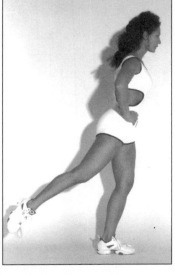

● Come up out of the lunge by pushing up with your back leg and extending it to the back, while lifting your body straight up. As you push up, really tighten the back of the leg, especially the buttocks, and straighten both legs.

● Bring the legs together again, ready to start your next repetition with the other leg.

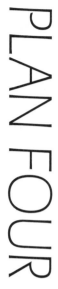

PLAN FOUR

TRAINER'S TIPS

▶ The important thing here is to really lengthen the front leg as you extend it forward. Feel as if your leg is moving away from your body, so that when you land into your lunge the front knee is directly on top of the ankle.

▶ As you come up from the lunge, really concentrate on keeping the body upright rather than leaning forward to help you get up. Your body needs to lift straight up so that you can retain control of the back leg extension.

● Do 16 repetitions with alternate legs, giving a total of 8 lunges on each leg. If you feel you can do more, then go for it!

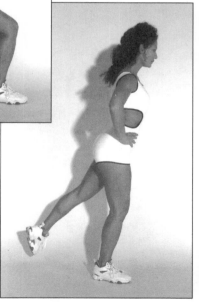

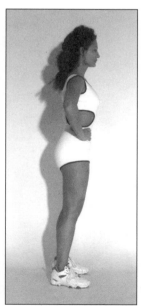

BUTT KICKER

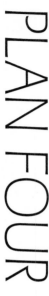

PLAN FOUR

This one tightens the buttocks and hamstrings. Placing a towel under your body, just near your belly-button and directly above your hip bones, will help you maintain a flat back for the duration of the exercise.

● Lie face down on the floor. To find the correct position for the towel, place your hands at the sides of your hips. The curved bones that you can feel on your sides are your hip bones, so make sure you place the towel above these to help flatten your back. Placing the towel too far down toward your thighs will have the opposite effect of increasing the curve in your low back as you perform the exercise.

● Now rest your head on your hands. Pull your abdomen up away from the towel as you raise one knee off the floor a little and bring your heel toward your buttocks, without arching your low back. How far you can lift the knee off the floor depends on how flat you can maintain your low back.

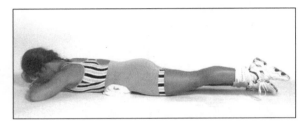

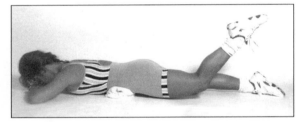

● Straighten the leg, keeping the knee off the floor, and follow straight through with your next repetition by bringing the heel toward your buttocks again. Aim to complete 8–10 repetitions before repeating with the other leg.

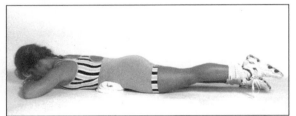

TRAINER'S TIPS

▶ Lifting your abdomen away from the towel will help keep the movement in the buttocks and hamstrings and prevent the back from arching.

▶ If you cannot keep the knee off the floor and your abdomen lifted for the duration of your repetitions, take a very short break by bringing the leg down to the floor, then reposition the leg for the next repetition.

Well done! Don't forget to move on to the Winding Down section on page 81.

WINDING DOWN

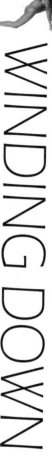

To those of you who have just completed your first workout, congratulations! You have taken the first step toward making some real changes in the way you look and feel. Most people would agree that after any exercise session we tend to feel much stronger, tighter and leaner. So, focus on these thoughts and really feel yourself getting better and stronger. Think about what you *have* achieved in your workout instead of dwelling on what you may not have done as well as you wished. From now on, it's going to get easier and the rewards will be more visible. The first step is the hardest, and you're already past that.

If you have been working out regularly and were able to get through your plan with ease while maintaining correct form throughout each repetition, then hats off to you as well. However, if you found yourself struggling with some of the exercises, then do go back and practise them before starting your next plan. Each plan focuses on certain skills, so be sure to master *each* exercise before heading on to the next plan.

Remember, the aim in Plan One is to move through the basic positions cleanly. The shoulder, hip, knee and ankle alignment will appear time and time again, which is why I cannot stress too highly the importance of acquiring the basic skills and working with them until they become second nature. So, always be confident in your technique and alignment before moving ahead. If you are already into Plan Four, I've got some variations for you later to help pump up the challenge.

Come on, let's start to wind down. Your body has just gone through a series of movements at varying joint angles, so you should be feeling nice and warm, which is why, in this cool-down section, we are going to concentrate on increasing flexibility.

Unlike in Gearing Up, where the movement was more fluid and continuous, we are now going to hold the stretch positions for a minimum of 25–35 counts – and, in some cases, for even longer. As you do these stretches I want you to actually count out, 1 Mississippi, 2 Mississippi … and so on, so that you can begin to gain a sense of how long 25 or 35 seconds really is. It is in this part of the program that you can really make improvements in your flexibility. So many people think it's enough just to do the toning exercises. But if you are to have the best body proportions you are capable of achieving, then you also need to have good overall flexibility. You want to make a difference to the shape of your buttocks and thighs? Right? Well, your range of movement – in other words, how far your muscles can lengthen and shorten – will greatly affect the look and shape of your buttocks and legs. We can't expect to utilize these greater ranges of movement if we do not stretch toward the limits of those ranges?

Makes sense? Right, so let's stretch.

WINDING DOWN

Note: It's important to know how to correctly stretch a muscle after practising the types of positions and methods used in this program. Here, we are primarily using the passive method of stretching where you get into the final position and hold – NO BOUNCING! Bouncing back and forth, even with control, is counter productive to our aim.

To get the maximum benefits out of each stretch, go into the position and then move further into the position until you feel tension in the muscle group you are stretching. Hold for the recommended number of counts or until you feel sufficiently stretched. If the tension eases, just move further into the stretch, then continue to hold. The less you force the position and just hold to where you are capable of holding, the more effective your stretch will be and you'll avoid injuring the muscle. Another tip is to breathe out when increasing the range of your stretch since this relaxes the body.

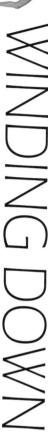

SIDE LUNGE STRETCH

In this stretch we want to get to the hamstrings and inner thighs. If you keep your abdomen lifted, you should have no problem with your balance, leaving you free to focus on the actual stretch.

● Stand with knees shoulder-width apart, resting both hands on your left thigh, well above the knee.

● Bend the left knee and, as you do so, straighten the right leg, pressing the hips back and leaning your upper body just a bit toward the left leg until you feel some tension in the hamstrings and inner thigh of the right leg. Hold and start counting slowly for 25–35 seconds.

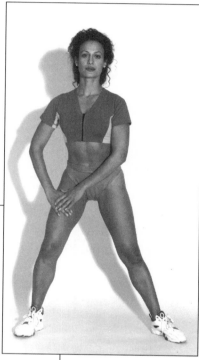

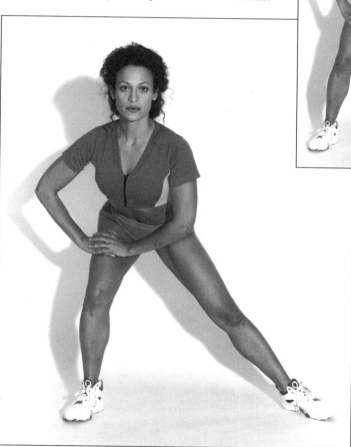

● Repeat to the other side by bending the right knee and straightening the left leg, making sure you rest your hands well above the right knee.

WINDING DOWN

WINDING DOWN

QUAD/HAMSTRING ELONGATION

Here we are going to stretch both the front and back of the thighs. The position of your low back will determine how successful you are in isolating the specific muscles, so don't let it arch. Use a chair for extra support, but remember, your lifted abdomen is going to act as your main support.

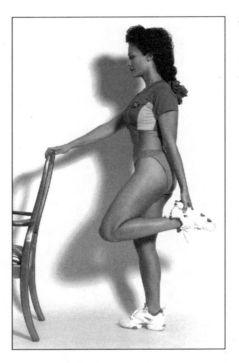

● Rest your right hand lightly on the back of the chair and shift your weight onto your right leg. Reach your left hand back and bring the heel of the left foot up to your left hand.

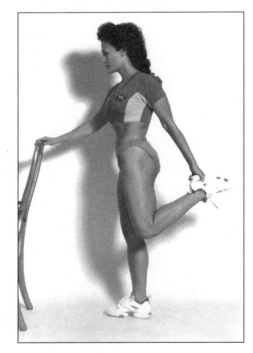

● The sequence for this stretch is very specific. So, hold the left heel and, lifting your abdomen, press the left knee back, without bringing the heel toward your buttocks. Once you have fully opened the front of the left thigh, you can then bring your heel toward your buttocks. Hold for a slow count of 25–30 seconds, maintaining your position, until you feel the tightness of the stretch ease a little.

● If you have pressed your knee back and fully opened the hip correctly, the heel will not be able to fully reach your buttocks, and you should feel a complete stretch in the front of the thigh.

● Now let's do the other side.

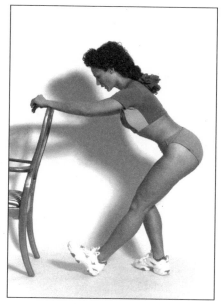

The hamstring part of this stretch is in two stages. For the first stage, have both hands resting on the back of the chair. You are going to straighten the left leg fully and sit back on your right leg with the right knee bent, all the while making sure you KEEP YOUR BACK FLAT.

- So, press your weight back onto your right leg, while straightening the left leg and flexing the left foot. Sit back until you feel a tightness in the back of the left leg and hold. Since the hamstrings tend to be tight, let's hold for 30–40 counts, starting 1 Mississippi, 2 Mississippi … Should you bend your upper body forward, be sure to bend from the hip (top of the thigh) so that the back remains flat.

- Let's repeat to the other side. Come on, hang in there for the full count. Your legs will thank you!

- OK, so you felt a stretch, but maybe it wasn't much of a stretch. If this is the case, you might like to move on to this more intense hamstring stretch. Turn the chair side on. Extend one leg on the arm or seat of the chair. Your back is upright and your abdomen is in and up. If you need to increase the stretch, bring your body forward by leading with your belly-button – avoid letting your body collapse forward. Again, hold for 30–40 counts.

- It may appear that not much is happening, but the back of the extended leg should feel longer as the tension eases, so continue to bend forward for the duration of the stretch. Don't forget to stretch the other leg.

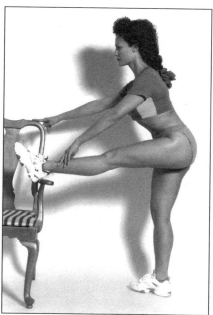

WINDING DOWN

8 5

THIGH STRETCHER

Right, let's stretch out the top of the thighs.

● Start with one knee down on the floor and the other leg bent in front with foot flat on the floor. Make sure the front leg is extended sufficiently, with the ankle ahead of the knee, so that as you move forward into position the front knee ends up directly on top of the ankle at a 90-degree angle.

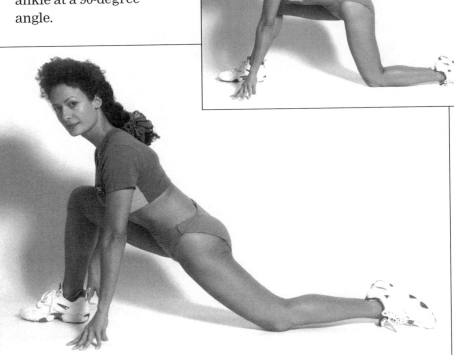

● Slowly press the top of the thigh of your back leg forward toward the floor, so that the front of the thigh feels very long, especially at the top (hip joint). Hold for 30–40 counts, always ensuring you hold to the point of tightness not pain.

● Repeat on the other side.

WINDING DOWN

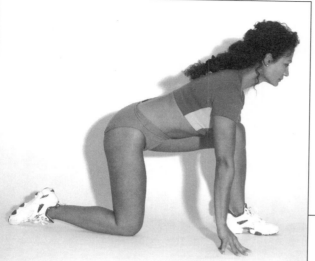

ON THE RACK

WINDING DOWN

This is a really great stretch for the low back and hamstrings, so try to remain in it for the full count.

● Your back knee is on the floor and your front leg is bent with the knee directly on top of the ankle.

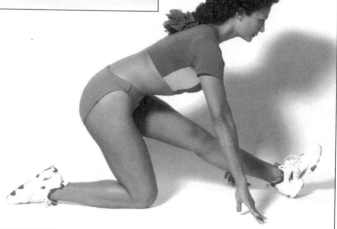

● From here you are going to move your weight back, making sure your weight does not fall directly on the kneecap of the supporting leg, but just below it. So, take care not not to sit on the back knee. The hips remain square, so that both hips maintain the same relationship to the leg on either side and neither leg is further forward from the hip than the other.

● Lift your abdomen as you straighten the front knee and move your weight back, taking care *not* to sit on your back leg. Continue to lift your bellybutton up and over toward your extended knee. Try to hold this stretch for 25–35 counts.

● Repeat on the other side.

8 7

WINDING DOWN

REACH OVER

Here we get to stretch a number of muscle groups – the back, the side of the waist, the inner thigh of the bent leg and the hamstring of the straight leg.

● Sit up tall with one leg extended. The other leg is bent, *with foot toward the centre of your body*. Try not to let your pelvis and stomach area collapse. Instead, sit up high on your pelvis and feel the lift in your torso.

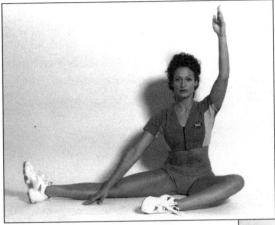

● Keeping your torso lifted, first reach one arm up and then over toward the extended leg. Keep your shoulders open and really try to maintain that lifted feeling throughout your body. Hold for a count of 20–30.

● Now, still maintaining the lift in your torso, bring both shoulders parallel to the floor as you lift your abdomen toward your knee and place your hands to either side of your extended leg. Once in position, try to melt into the floor and keep the bent leg relaxed. Hold for another 20–30 counts.

● Repeat the whole sequence to the other side.

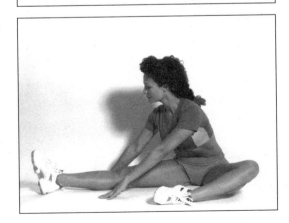

ROTATION REACH

This one stretches the hamstrings and the rotators – the small group of muscles that lie deep under the buttocks and which are responsible for your turn-out.

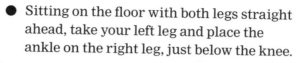

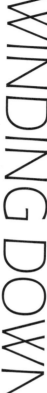

● Sitting on the floor with both legs straight ahead, take your left leg and place the ankle on the right leg, just below the knee.

● Reach straight up and take your arms, along with the whole of your upper body, up and over your legs toward the floor. Rest your hands on your leg or on the floor, whichever is more comfortable, so that you can relax into the stretch. Hold for 20–30 counts. Continue lifting your belly-button so that the whole of your upper body from the waist up is reaching over the leg.

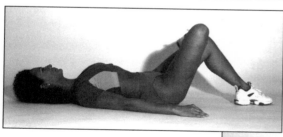

● If your hamstrings and rotators are very tight, you might find it difficult to hold this position. If so, try doing this stretch lying on your back. The leg positioning is the same. Just pull both legs toward you and hold for 20–30 counts.

Stay with me, we're almost done ...

89

WAIST STRETCH

WINDING DOWN

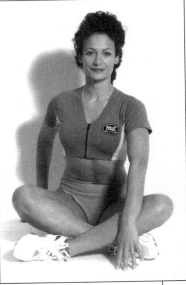

● Sit up with legs comfortably crossed. Maintaining a lift in your abdomen, place one hand in front of your legs and the other hand behind you.

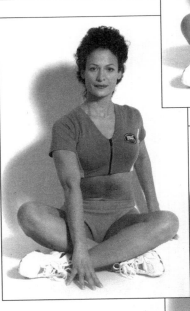

● Keeping your shoulders and abdomen lifted, twist from the waist as you turn your upper body and look past your shoulder. *Stay lifted throughout the movement* and hold for 20–30 counts.

● Slowly return to the centre and repeat to the other side.

HEAD STRETCH

Although we are actually stretching the neck, I call this one the head stretch because this position offers a good opportunity to close your eyes and quieten your mind.

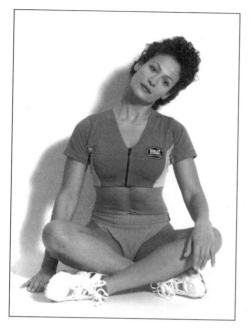

- Still sitting with legs crossed and torso lifted, allow your head to fall gently to one side, aiming the ear toward the shoulder while letting the opposite shoulder fall toward the floor. Hold for 20–25 counts.

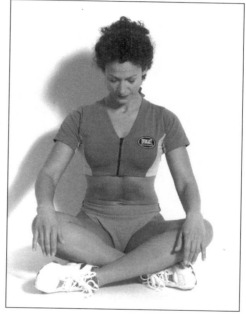

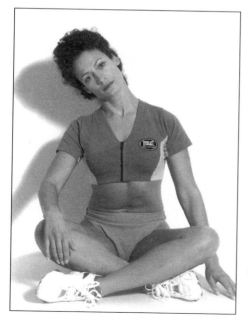

- Let your head slowly roll forward. Stay here and relax your shoulders for 20 counts.

- Now, let the head roll slowly to the other side so that the ear is aiming toward the shoulder. Hold for a 20–25 second count.

- If your shoulders or neck still feel really tight, go through this sequence again.

WINDING DOWN

91

WINDING DOWN

TOTAL FOLD-OVER

Here's a really comfortable position that will allow you to fully stretch your back.

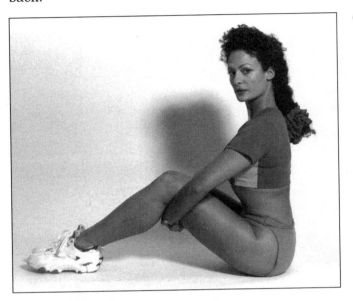

● Sit up tall with knees bent. Place both arms under your knees, with each hand clasping the opposite arm.

● Slowly start to fold your upper body over your legs by lifting from your chest first and then allowing the head and shoulders to relax over the legs. Carry the movement through the arms and into the hands so that your arms extend and your hands are on the floor. Let your legs

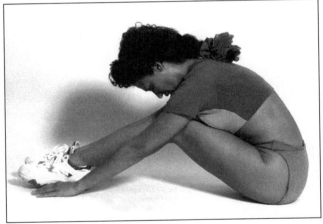

extend slightly but do not straighten them completely. Take some nice long breaths and feel yourself sinking toward your legs, but keep the back rounded. Ahhhhh! Doesn't that feel good? In fact, it feels so good, let's stay here for a count of 40. Take longer, if you need to – just stay here and relax.

We're almost home …

COMPLETE LEG STRETCH

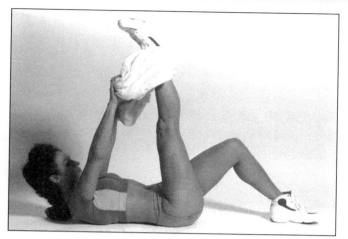

A great one for the hamstrings and low back.

● Grab a towel and lie back on the floor with knees bent. Raise one leg and place the towel round your ankle and lower calf area.

● Relax your head, neck and shoulders into the floor. Gently bring the towel toward you and hold the position at the first sign of mild tension.

● Keep your head, neck and shoulders relaxed. Breathe out and, as you do so, allow the leg to fall further into the stretch. Keep deepening your breathing and your stretch for a 30–40 second count.

● Repeat on the other side.

Just one more to go …

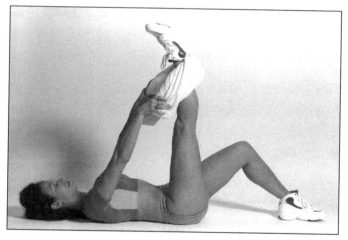

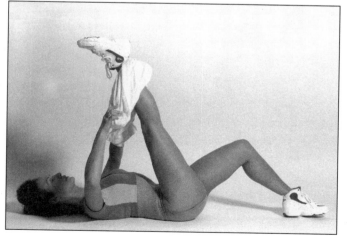

WINDING DOWN

WINDING DOWN

THIGH FOLD-OVER

This last one is for the buttocks and outer thighs.

● Still lying on your back, extend both legs. Let your body completely relax into the floor, releasing all the tension in your shoulders, neck, face and torso. Bend your left leg, lifting it off the floor, and take hold of the outside of the leg with your right arm, just above the knee. Your left arm is outstretched on the floor, away from your body.

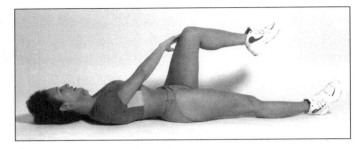

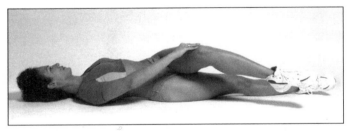

● Fold the left leg over the right leg, making sure BOTH shoulders remain on the floor. Take long breaths and hold for 30–40 counts.

● Repeat to the other side.

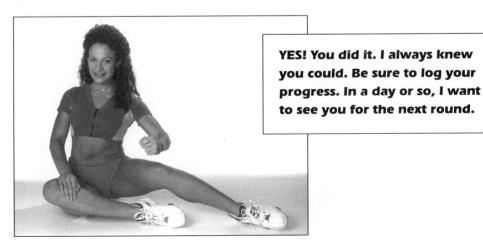

YES! You did it. I always knew you could. Be sure to log your progress. In a day or so, I want to see you for the next round.

9 4

CHAPTER FOUR

The Bottom Line Break

So, you've completed all four plans. Congratulations! It's probably about six to eight weeks since you began your Bottom Line program. Remember, healthy eating is an integral part of the formula in our fitness equation, so I hope you've also been following the healthy eating advice in chapter 5. Your legs are now stronger and leaner and your posture is much improved. Getting to this point was not easy. It required a great deal of discipline, and you should be proud of your achievements.

Increasing the challenge

Well, it doesn't end here. In order to maintain the benefits you have gained and to continue progressing you need to change the stimulus to your muscles. In other words, you need to change the way you perform an exercise. So why is this necessary?

After a while, when a muscle becomes accustomed to a certain stimulus, its response to that stimulus diminishes or stops altogether. Imagine you were in an environment where each day at noon you heard a loud scream. At first you'd be quite startled, but as the days went by you'd gradually start to get accustomed to the scream. After a week or so, you'd probably hardly notice it. This is similar to what happens with the muscles if we continue to do the same exercises in the same way over and over again. That's why in this chapter I've come up with some new challenges and variations on existing exercises to prevent you from experiencing any plateaus or diminished results.

First, you'll find three completely new exercises involving partner work to provide added incentive to your workout. Work with each other, challenge each other, spur each other on, and you'll be amazed at how much you can achieve. Next, I have then taken some of my favourite exercises – and yours too I hope – from this Bottom Line program and given them a different dimension. In some cases, I've extended the number of counts so that you

9 5

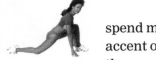

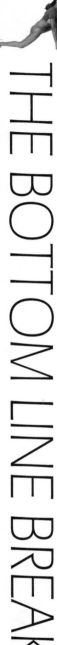

THE BOTTOM LINE BREAK

spend more time in certain key positions. In others, I have changed the accent or emphasis in the move or asked you to repeat specific phases within the overall sequence.

Using the variations to best effect

There are several ways that you can incorporate these variations into your program to help you stay challenged and focused. The first is to take one of the four existing plans and substitute two or three of the exercises with the relevant variations in this chapter. For instance, in Plan One you could substitute the Straight Squat, Power Legs and Easy Chair Extensions with the modified versions on the following pages.

Alternatively, you could simply select several exercises from this chapter to create your own workout. If you choose this option, then make sure you adhere to the following guidelines to maximize the benefits from your workout.

▶ Always begin by doing the warm-up movements in the Gearing Up section (see pages 21–32). This is essential if you are to get the most out of your workout and avoid injury.

▶ Vary your choices so that you achieve a balanced workout and avoid working the same muscle groups over and over again. On one particular day you might choose to focus on buttocks, along with some outer thigh work. So, formulate a plan and avoid making arbitrary selections.

▶ Always finish your session with some stretching (see Winding Down, pages 81–94). This is the optimum time to work on increasing your flexibility and it also helps to prevent any soreness you may experience over the next few days.

Following these simple guidelines will ensure you get the best out of your workout and allow you to re-create your own program over and over. If you want a real challenge, you could combine a selection of exercises from each plan and put together your own killer workout! The options are endless. Just remember to follow the above guidelines. Use the Training Log on page 119 to keep track of the exercises you've been working on and to chart your ongoing progress. Keeping a written record in this way is a great motivator to spur you on to further challenges.

You've made great progress so far. Come on, let's move into the variations and put together our next workout.

TWIN SEATS

This is the first of three exercises involving partner work. Here you are going to challenge your partner as to who can land more softly and with knees directly over the ankles.

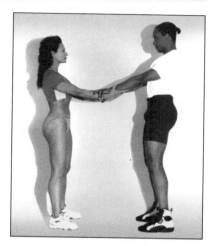

- Stand face to face with your partner, holding each other's arms lightly, just above the wrists. Arms are slightly extended so that you are not standing too close to each other.

- Bend your knees and sit back into your squat position, taking care to use your abdomen for balance and not to rely on the other person to hold you up – unless of course this was mutually agreed before you began the exercise!

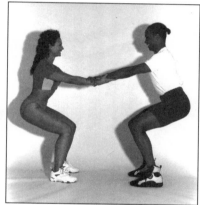

- From here you are going to jump, so count down 3...2...1 and spring into the air simultaneously with your partner, lifting your body and springing high enough to allow your legs to straighten fully. Land *smoothly*, through your legs, making sure you bend the knees as you land. Stand up straight again, then go down in to the squat and cue each other to go into the next jump.

- Go for 4 repetitions in as controlled a fashion as you can – or more if you are both up to the challenge. Try to get a bit higher in the air on each jump.

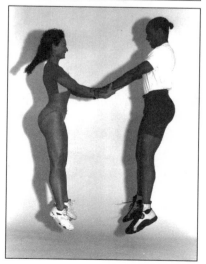

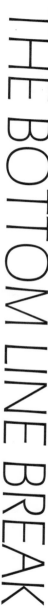

THE BOTTOM LINE BREAK

THE BOTTOM LINE BREAK

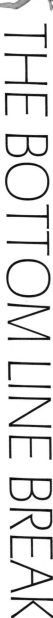

INNER/OUTER LIMITS

In this exercise, one of you is going to push outward with the legs while the other partner will try to resist this by pushing inward. This really hits the inner and outer thighs.

● Sit on the floor with your legs inside your partner's. Gently hold onto each other's arms at or above the elbows. You are going to push outward with your legs while your partner will try to keep your legs in by pressing inward. Cue each other and begin counting 1...2...3...4...5...6...7...8. Lift your abdomen as you press the legs and *do not allow your partner to sink –* make them sit up tall. If 8 counts is too long, then just aim to hold for 4 counts at first. Or, if you feel you can do more, aim to hold for longer if you wish.

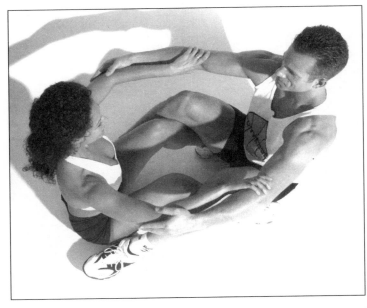

● Open the legs a little wider and push and press again for at least the same count, whether it's 4, 8 or 16. Open the legs even wider and press again for the same count.

● After pressing and holding in at least three different leg-width positions, switch legs, so that your partner's legs are now inside yours and your roles are reversed. Repeat the exercise, holding for the same number of counts as before in each position. Work up to holding in each of the three positions for a count of 16.

● Really challenge each other and have fun!

GRAVITY DEFIER

This one works the hamstrings intensely. You will require some form of box that you'll be able to lean on at the end of your repetitions if necessary. Your partner is going to hold your legs to help support you while you complete the exercise. Then you can switch positions to let your partner do the exercise.

- Kneel in front of the box. If you find kneeling uncomfortable, place a pillow or towel under your knees. Your partner is holding your legs down just above the ankles.

- As your partner holds your legs down, make a really strong effort to lift your abdomen and allow your body, from your knees to the top of your head, to move forward in one solid unit. Remember, I said move forward, NOT FALL FORWARD. Try to maintain control as the body continues to go forward.

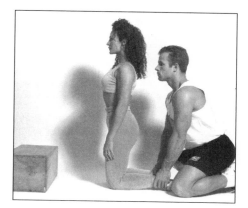

- Have your hands prepared, ready to be lifted in front, so that as soon as you can no longer maintain control you can place them on your support box to prevent yourself from falling.

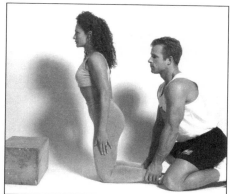

- Depending on how you feel after the first repetition, you may wish to take a break and let your partner have a go. Start with just 2–4 repetitions at first, ultimately aiming to complete 8, holding each attempt for as long as you can.

- This is a tough one, so cheer your partner on.

Let's now move on to some variations on existing exercises from Plans One to Four.

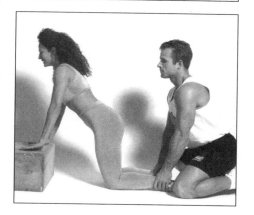

STRAIGHT SQUAT

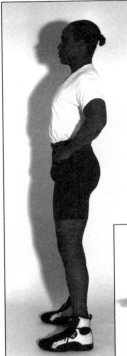

THE BOTTOM LINE BREAK

In this variation we are going to stay down in the squat a little longer, so be sure to keep your knees over your ankles.

- Go down into your squat position on counts 1...2...3. Really squeeze your buttocks to come up on count 4.

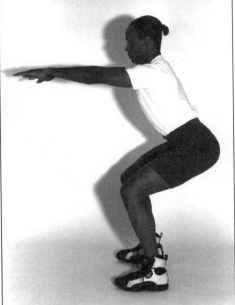

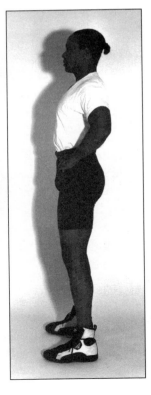

- Repeat 4–8 times. Once you feel as if your body is just giving in to gravity and you can no longer feel lifted as you descend, take a break.

POWER LEGS

Here we will be spending more time with the legs apart in the descending phase of this exercise, so please keep that front knee directly above the ankle.

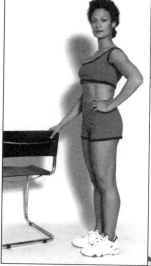

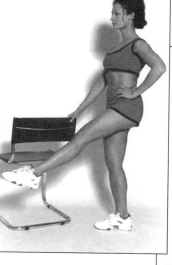

● Stand up straight on count 1, lunge 2...3...4. Come back up and bring feet together on 5...6.

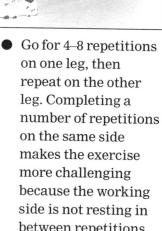

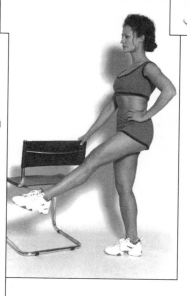

● Go for 4–8 repetitions on one leg, then repeat on the other leg. Completing a number of repetitions on the same side makes the exercise more challenging because the working side is not resting in between repetitions.

THE BOTTOM LINE BREAK

THE BOTTOM LINE BREAK

EASY CHAIR EXTENSIONS

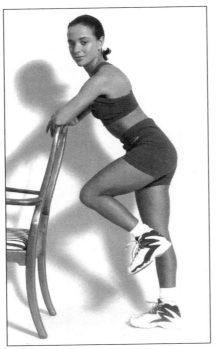

In this one we are going to keep the leg extended for an extra count, so keep your low back firmly in place.

● Bring the knee up on count 1, straighten the leg on 2, squeeze the buttocks and lengthen the leg further 3...4. Go right into your next repetition, bringing the knee up again on count 1 and extending the leg 2...3...4. The working leg does not come back to the floor until you have completed 6–8 repetitions, so your supporting leg and abdomen will act as your main support.

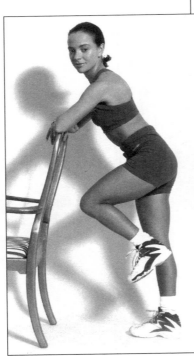

● Repeat with the other leg. Remember to do an equal number of repetitions on each leg. By now, you know that your low back has to stay firmly in place, regardless of how far back you push the leg.

OUTER THIGH ERASER

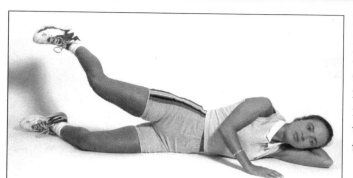

Here we are going to maintain the leg in the lifted position for the duration of our repetitions. This will increase the work for the hip on that side of the body.

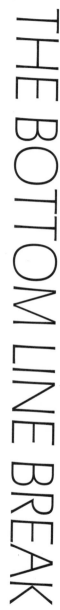

THE BOTTOM LINE BREAK

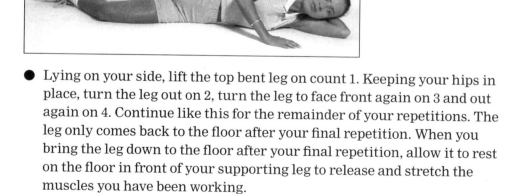

- Lying on your side, lift the top bent leg on count 1. Keeping your hips in place, turn the leg out on 2, turn the leg to face front again on 3 and out again on 4. Continue like this for the remainder of your repetitions. The leg only comes back to the floor after your final repetition. When you bring the leg down to the floor after your final repetition, allow it to rest on the floor in front of your supporting leg to release and stretch the muscles you have been working.

- Do 4–8 repetitions – or more if you feel able!

- Roll over and repeat with the other leg. Be sure to do an equal number of repetitions on each leg.

THE BOTTOM LINE BREAK

COMPLETE LEG

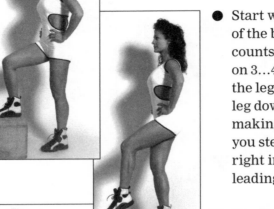

In this variation, after lifting the knee and straightening the leg back we are going to bring the knee in again and extend the leg back for a second time.

- Start with one foot up on the centre of the box. Bring the knee up on counts 1...2. Same leg presses back on 3...4. Knee up again on 5...6. Press the leg back again on 7...8. Bring the leg down to the floor on 9...10, making sure you bend the knee as you step down. Straighten up and go right into your next repetition, leading with the same leg.

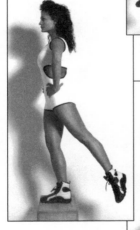

- The key here is to avoid swinging the leg. Instead, aim to control its movement and placement, all the while pulling the abdomen up. This is a lot of effort for the working side of the body, so start with a low number of repetitions and aim for good form. Try 4 complete cycles, then try one more.

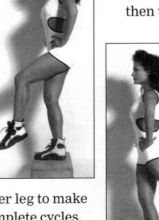

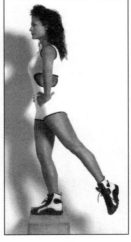

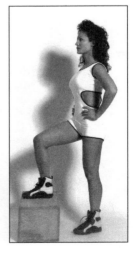

- Repeat on the other leg to make it up to 8 or 10 complete cycles.

LATERAL LEG LIFTER

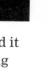

Here, once the leg is lifted we are going to hold it up for 2 counts before returning to the starting position.

● Start in the basic squat position. Lift leg up on count 1, hold or lift a bit higher if you can on 2...3. Slowly bring the leg down and go into your squat on count 4. Repeat, lifting the other leg.

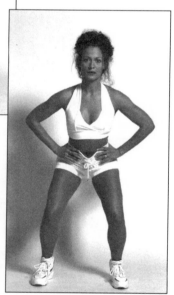

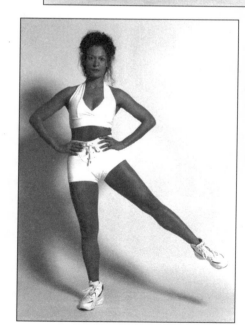

● Balance is everything in this one, so really feel those abdominal muscles helping you to stay upright. Go for 8 repetitions with alternate legs.

THE BOTTOM LINE BREAK

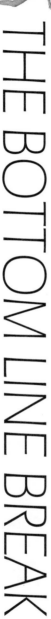

THE BOTTOM LINE BREAK

THREE POINT LUNGE

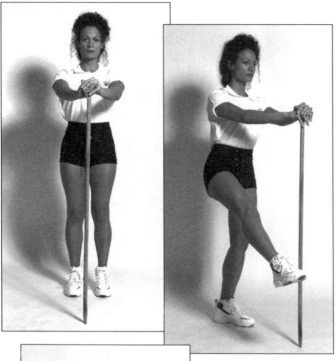

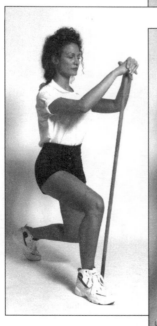

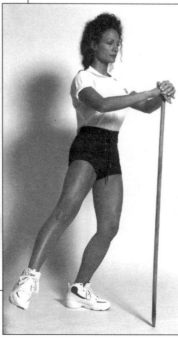

In this variation we are going to add a spring in between each position – just high enough to allow you to straighten your legs and point your toes. Be sure to land with knees bending softly as soon as you make contact with the floor. Adding a spring will bring your heart rate up, so try to keep your breathing smooth and regular and listen to your jumps.

● Start with your pole comfortably in front of you. Leg reaches forward on count 1. Go down into the lunge on 2. Hop up and reach the leg out to the side on 3. Go down into your squat on 4. Hop up and swing leg to the back on 5. Go down into a back lunge on 6. Hop up and bring legs together 7...8.

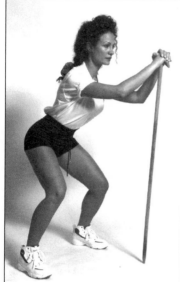

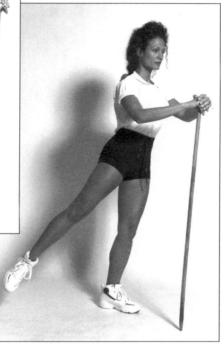

● Try to go through a full series of springs once on each side. When you feel ready to add more, go for 4–8 repetitions on alternate sides. Yeah!

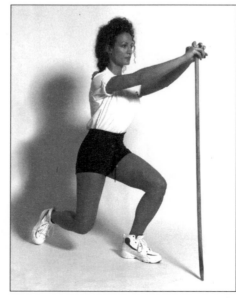

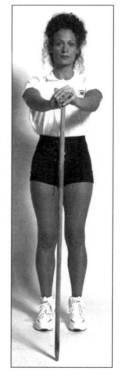

THE BOTTOM LINE BREAK

THE BOTTOM LINE BREAK

BUTT ROTATOR

Here, once the knee is fully turned out we are going lift the leg back and up just a little before bringing it down. Remember how important it is to maintain a straight back when resting on your forearms and knees.

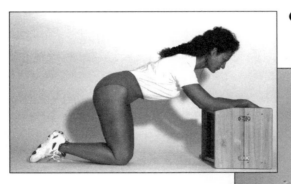

● Start on your knees with forearms resting on your support box, heels together.

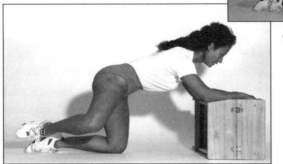

● Keeping the heels together, turn out the knee on count 1. Maintaining the turn-out, lift the leg away from your bottom just a bit on 2. Bring the knee down on 3, so that the heels are together again but the knee is just off the floor. Release the turn-out on 4, then go straight into your next repetition. The knee does not come down to the floor until you have completed your repetitions.

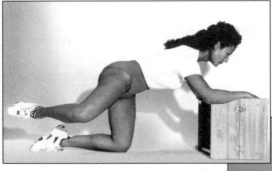

● Aim for 8 repetitions, then repeat with the other leg. Be sure to maintain a flat back throughout.

BUTT KICKER

In this variation we're going to spend more time with the leg off the floor to really work the hamstrings.

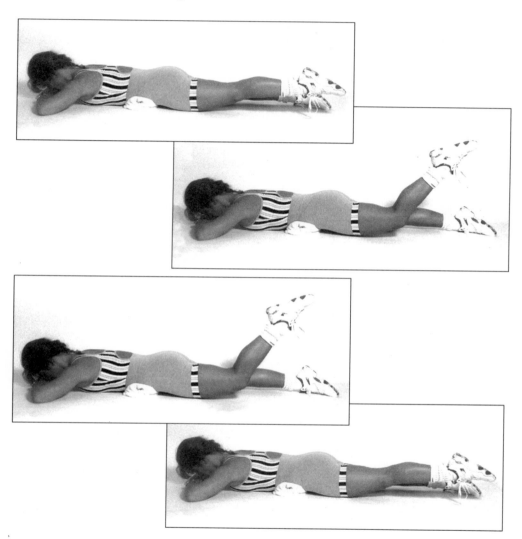

● Keeping your abdomen up, lift the leg on 1, pull the heel in toward the buttocks on 2, pull the heel in again on 3, straighten the leg on 4 without letting the knee drop to the floor.

● The leg does not touch the floor again until you have completed at least 4 sets of the cycle. If you feel you can get at least one more in, then DO IT! Remember to do the same number of sets on the other leg.

1 0 9

CHAPTER FIVE

Your Guide to Healthy Eating

You have taken the decision to improve your body shape through exercise. That's great. Exercise can make a dramatic difference to the way you look and feel, and if you've already started working your way through the Bottom Line program then I'm sure you will have noticed some significant improvements in your health and wellbeing. Your body is becoming stronger each day, your energy level is increasing and your muscles are starting to shape up. Once you've taken the first step toward a leaner, fitter and healthier body, you'll find the benefits are so great that you will want to do everything you possibly can to maintain your body in tip-top condition and maximize the benefits from your Bottom Line program. And that's where healthy eating comes into the equation.

EATING FOR HEALTH

Healthy eating combined with regular exercise is the best way toward a healthy lifestyle, so the aim of this chapter is to provide you with some basic nutritional tips and guidelines to complement your program of exercise. If you need to lose weight, then the advice in this chapter will set you on the right path. All food provides us with energy in the form of calories, and if we eat more calories than the body needs, then the excess will be stored in the body as fat. Monitoring our food intake, making the right choices in the type of foods we eat and eating them in the right proportions will, together with our exercise program, help us achieve a weight with which we feel comfortable, one that is realistic to maintain. It will also ensure that we obtain a balanced intake of essential nutrients for health.

Let's start by looking at some fundamental facts about carbohydrate, protein and fat, the essential energy-giving foods.

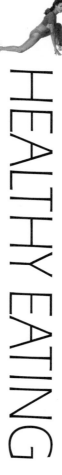

Carbohydrate – good or bad?

Carbohydrate is the basic building block for energy and breaks down into two categories – simple and complex.

Simple carbohydrates are found in refined sugar and sugary foods such as candy or sweets, cakes, biscuits, juices, syrups and soft drinks. These foods offer little in the way of nutritional value and should be kept to a minimum in a healthy diet.

Complex carbohydrates, on the other hand, do not contain as much highly refined sugar and consist of starchy foods such as grains (which include bread, rice, potatoes, pasta, cereal), pulses (legumes), nuts and some vegetables. The unrefined carbohydrates offer a greater nutritional value than the refined versions and are also rich in fibre, a wonderful substance that adds bulk to your diet and helps fill you up. Fibre-rich foods help you eliminate waste more efficiently as well as helping to reduce your cholesterol level.

Particularly good sources of fibre are vegetables such as spinach and lettuce, pulses (legumes) and beans such as lentils, kidney beans and chick peas. Fresh fruit, although not generally considered a complex carbohydrate, also contains plenty of fibre, especially fruit where the skin can be eaten such as apples, peaches and pears.

Although both types of carbohydrates provide energy, simple carbohydrates are quickly digested by the body. Complex carbohydrates, however, are absorbed more slowly and therefore provide the body with a longer lasting and more valuable source of energy, which is particularly important if you exercise regularly. Complex carbohydrates also help keep the metabolism – that's the rate at which we burn calories – fuelled and prevent the drops in blood sugar levels that can lead to sugar cravings. Aim to eat around four ounces (100 grams) to 10 ounces (275 grams) of complex carbohydrates per day, and choose wholegrain rather than refined carbohydrates. If you wish, you could break this down into several small servings throughout the day. For instance, a small serving could be a palmful of rice or almonds.

Protein – food for muscles

Protein is another terrific energy provider and, most important, an essential building block for muscles. It can be utilized more efficiently than any other substance in the body, except for water. Protein is broken down in the body much more slowly than carbohydrate. In fact, it takes about 30 days for protein to be completely broken down in the digestive system and have a measurable impact on increasing your body weight or your muscle mass.

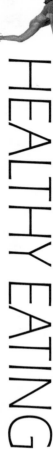

HEALTHY EATING

Generally, we need around eight ounces (225 grams) of protein per day, but this varies according to the individual and their specific body weight. Since both exercise and stress accelerate the body's utilization of protein, the more physical activity you undertake and the greater your level of stress, the more protein you will need.

Think of protein as food for your muscles that helps them to get bigger and stronger. The leaner the protein, the leaner the body, so bear this in mind when making your protein selections and choose low-fat sources where possible. Egg whites, turkey breast or chicken (white meat only) and fish are all high in protein and low in fat, but remember to bake or grill (broil) these foods in preference to frying..

Beans and pulses (legumes) such as kidney beans and chick peas also contain protein but need to be combined with grains to form 'complete' proteins. This way, they form good alternatives to meat and contain a lot less fat. They are versatile foods which can be easily mixed with rice, pasta and salad to form a tasty and nutrition-packed meal. If you don't have time to soak the dried varieties, use canned ones. Just rinse the beans well, mix in some garlic, add a little salt and pepper and add to any salad, pasta or entrée.

Get your fats right

Let me explain a little about fats. Fats can creep up on you without warning. A little fat can add a lot of calories, since fat contains twice the calories of carbohydrate or protein – so proceed cautiously! The fat we eat is easily stored by the body. What's more, if we consume excess amounts of carbohydrates and alcohol, these will ultimately be converted to and stored in the body as fat and lead to weight gain. Eating too much of the wrong kind of fat can also increase our risk of heart disease and other health problems.

However, we all need to eat a small amount of fat since it has several important functions. Fat acts as an insulator to help us retain body heat and it cushions our internal organs, keeping them in place and protecting them from damage. It helps the body absorb the fat-soluble vitamins A, D, E and K. Since fat is broken down slowly in the digestive system, it keeps the metabolism fuelled during prolonged bouts of exercise. Certain essential fatty acids which are important for health cannot be made by the body and so have to be obtained from our food. The fats found in fish oils are particularly beneficial in helping to protect against heart disease.

So, we do need some fat, but it should form only a small proportion of our total food intake. Aim to minimize your fat intake and select the right kind of fat. Choose unsaturated fats in preference to saturated ones. Unsaturated fats are usually liquid or soft at room temperature, e.g. soft margarine, vegetable oil and olive oil, whereas saturated fats are solid, e.g. butter, lard, hard margarine. Avoid eating large quantities of saturated fats, since these can raise cholesterol levels.

To cut down on the fat, try to bake or grill (broil) foods instead of frying. Choose lean cuts of meat, trim off all visible fat and remove all skin from chicken or turkey before cooking. And don't forget that many foods such as cakes, biscuits and muffins also contain large amounts of fat.

EATING, EXERCISE AND WEIGHT CONTROL

Keeping your weight under control will not only help you achieve a more attractive body shape, but it can also reduce your risk of suffering serious health problems. Obesity is a leading contributor to many diseases such as diabetes, high cholesterol, high blood pressure, heart attack – even arthritis – as well as affecting your self-esteem. Imagine carrying around a five-pound (two-kilogram) bag of potatoes with you all day and every day. Try it for just ten minutes and you'll see how much effort is required. Five extra pounds alone can put a strain not only on your heart but also on your bones, organs and muscles, so just think of the amount of damage that could be done if you were substantially overweight.

Exercise and portion control are the two chief factors in weight control. To lose weight, therefore, you need to cut out the excess calories and step up your activity level to help pump up your metabolic rate. If you were simply to decrease your intake of food without exercising, or if you were to drastically reduce your calorie intake, your metabolic rate would slow down and your body would become less efficient at burning calories. This is why crash diets don't work in the long term. In the end you would simply regain all your lost weight – and possibly more. Many people spend a lifetime on the diet rollercoaster.

Assess your eating habits

There are many reasons why people overeat, so understanding why you eat is another important factor in weight control. People tend to eat if they are anxious, depressed, bored, or simply because they always have something to eat at that particular time of day. Instead of just eating out of habit at set times of the day such as at lunch-time, tea-time and so on, try to train yourself to eat only when you are hungry.

113

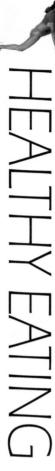

HEALTHY EATING

It's extremely helpful to keep a food diary (see page 120), particularly when starting out on a new eating regime. Recording everything you eat each day, along with the time of day and the reason, and noting down any mood swings you may experience will give you an overall picture of your eating habits and enable you to easily identify any 'wasted' calories or problem foods. It will also help you to establish if you are eating a varied and balanced intake of foods.

Take it slowly

Before starting any new eating regime, ask yourself if you are ready to make some changes. It's important to make a real commitment before you start. And when you start, take it one step at a time. So many people take an 'all or nothing' approach by making too many drastic changes too soon and simply end up slipping back into their old habits.

Rule number one, therefore, is to set yourself small goals, and implement them one at a time. Don't forget to record them in your food diary. Constantly review your diary and see which foods you can substitute for which. For instance, you could start by choosing skimmed or semi-skimmed milk in preference to whole milk, using low-fat or fat-free dressings instead of regular dressings, or leaving out the egg yolks in an omelette. Cut out the butter on that bagel or roll, and use jam instead of cream cheese. Substitute mustard for mayonnaise. See how easy it can be. Just remember to make only one change at a time. Be imaginative and use herbs and spices for extra flavouring. Limit your intake of condiments and sauces as these can add on the calories.

For a quick and easy low-fat meal, try making a spinach and onion omelette using egg whites. Use a paper towel and a little oil or fat-free spray to wipe or spray the inside of a frying pan so that the eggs won't stick. Place four egg whites in the pan, add some chopped spinach (fresh or frozen) and some red or white onions. Wait until the eggs become firm and then fold the omelette in half. In about eight to ten minutes you will have a delicious and satisfying high-protein, low-fat entrée that can be eaten at any time of the day.

Control the portions

Get into the habit of monitoring your food portions – moderation is the key. Try eating your meals on a salad plate (side plate) instead of a dinner plate. This will help prevent you from overeating, provided you don't go back for seconds! When describing portions of food in your food diary, use visual terms such as a handful of pasta, three walnut sizes of rice, a half deck of cards of meat. You will be surprised to see what a difference it makes to keep track of these small changes. If you find yourself tempted to eat something you know you really shouldn't, just say to yourself 'I've had this before. I know what it tastes like. Is it really necessary – and worth it?' If you do find yourself giving into temptation, see it as just a small step back and resolve to get back on track as soon as possible. Remember, a small battle that does not go as planned does not mean you've lost the war.

Identify your problem foods

Almost everyone has their weak spots or favourite foods that once eaten can lead to uncontrollable cravings. To identify which foods, if any, affect you in this way, consider these two questions:

Which foods do I find that once I start eating them I can't stop?

What type of foods do I consume most often?

Answering these questions can help you single out specific problem foods so that you can take steps to avoid them where possible. For instance, when I go out to dinner I have trouble controlling my consumption of bread from the bread basket. So, *before* the bread has a chance to hit the table, I request that none be brought over. Or, if I'm dining with friends and I can't avoid having the bread basket on the table, I take the decision not to *start* eating it and place the basket out of reach. If you find yourself with an uncontrollable craving for a certain problem food, redirect your thought process by occupying yourself with some other activity. Do the laundry, pick up that book you've been meaning to start, brush your teeth, chew some gum or, better still, take a walk or do some other exercise. Exercise will make you feel better, you'll burn calories and be yet another step closer to your goal.

WHAT KIND OF PERSONA ARE YOU?

Broadly speaking, people fall into one of two categories – the low-carbohydrate persona or the low-fat persona. The low-carbohydrate persona is someone who craves carbohydrates and finds it relatively difficult to lose weight and/or who puts on weight easily because their body is not able to break down food easily and burn up calories. The low-fat persona, on the other hand, tends to find it easier to maintain their existing weight and/or does not put on weight easily. The type of persona you are can influence the type of foods you need to eat, so before making any changes to your eating habits, answer the simple questions on the next two pages:

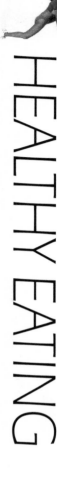

HEALTHY EATING

1. How many times a week do you exercise?

1	2	3	4	5	6	7
❑	❑	❑	❑	❑	❑	❑

2. Do you make an effort to eat low-fat foods?

ALWAYS	5	❑
USUALLY	4	❑
SOMETIMES	3	❑
RARELY	2	❑

3. Approximately how many servings of starchy food (bread, potatoes, etc.) do you eat each day?

MORE THAN 10	5	❑
8 – 10	4	❑
6 – 8	3	❑
4 – 6	2	❑
0 – 3	1	❑

4. Do you tend to work off calories easily? (Rate your answer on a scale of ten.)

YES   NO

1	2	3	4	5	6	7	8	9	10
❑	❑	❑	❑	❑	❑	❑	❑	❑	❑

5. How difficult is it for you to lose weight? (Rate your answer on a scale of ten.)

EASY   DIFFICULT

1	2	3	4	5	6	7	8	9	10
❑	❑	❑	❑	❑	❑	❑	❑	❑	❑

6. Do you feel constantly bloated and retain fluids easily? (Rate your answer on a scale of ten.)

NEVER   ALWAYS

1	2	3	4	5	6	7	8	9	10
❑	❑	❑	❑	❑	❑	❑	❑	❑	❑

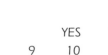

7. Do you think you eat very little but still can't lose weight? (Rate your answer on a scale of ten.)

NO   YES

1   2   3   4   5   6   7   8   9   10

☐   ☐   ☐   ☐   ☐   ☐   ☐   ☐   ☐   ☐

Now add up your scores:

If you scored 32 points or more, then you are considered to be a low-carbohydrate persona.

If you scored 31 points or less, then you are considered to be a low-fat persona.

Now, let's review the eating regimens for the two different personas.

The low-carbohydrate persona – what to eat

If you fall into this category and have been attempting to lose weight to no avail, try cutting down on the amount of starchy carbohydrates you eat such as bread, pasta and rice, and reduce your intake of fat. Aim to base your meals around raw, steamed or boiled vegetables, salads with low-fat or fat-free dressings, and lean protein. Egg whites, minced (ground) turkey or chicken (white meat only), beans and pulses (legumes) make good low-fat protein choices. So, instead of having a bowl of spaghetti, make a salad, adding just a little pasta, or try lentils with lots of fresh vegetables to take the focus off the carbohydrates. In addition, drink plenty of water each day.

Following these guidelines will help cleanse your system without leaving you hungry. At first you may experience some withdrawal symptoms, but these should last only a couple of weeks. So, stick it out, and not only will you feel more energized, but you'll also find that the excess weight starts to come off. Remember, the changes should be gradual. Don't forget to record them in your food diary.

The low-carbohydrate persona often finds it difficult to lose the last five to ten pounds (two to five kilos) of excess weight. If this happens, try gradually increasing your calorie intake or changing the proportions of foods you eat. Here's where you might want to increase your intake of carbohydrates by eating one or two extra slices of bread a day and cutting out one or two servings of protein. Try this for a week or so, and the increased calorie intake will raise your metabolism to help you burn off the excess calories, in the same way that exercise does. Some people find it helps to eat small meals or snacks throughout the day. This provides your body with a constant supply of fuel which helps to keep the metabolism running higher. For instance, you

HEALTHY EATING

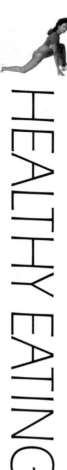

could 'graze' on protein snacks with a little bread during the day, then in the evening eat some vegetables and fruit to add fibre and bulk to your eating plan.

The low-fat persona – what to eat

The low-fat persona tends to be able to break down foods at a faster rate than the low-carbohydrate persona and therefore burns off the calories more easily. If you fall into this category, you can usually eat as many complex carbohydrates as you like, provided you control your intake of fat. Limit the protein to around six to eight ounces (175 to 225 grams) per day. To get a feel for this amount, think of it as two decks of cards or twice the size of the palm of your hand. Drink plenty of water each day. If you stick to these guidelines you should find it easy to control your weight and feel healthier for it. Again, incorporate any changes you make one at a time and don't forget to keep a record in your food diary.

STAY ACTIVE AND EAT HEALTHILY FOR LIFE

As you've learned in this chapter, regular exercise and moderation in your food intake are the two key factors for successful weight control, not just in the short term but for ever. So stick with it! Remember, everyone is different, so find the eating plan that suits you, one that you can comfortably maintain. Once you start to exercise regularly and consume the right kind of foods in the right quantities, your body will soon start to show the results. The bottom line is that if you keep this up you should reap the benefits for a lifetime.

THE BOTTOM LINE TRAINING LOG

Make several copies of the blank log so that you can continue to chart your progress, whichever plan you are following or when creating your own program. Remember to fill in your results immediately after your workout, as it is easy to forget later how much you have accomplished. Stick the log up in a highly visible place so you have a constant reminder of your progress.

NAME .... PLAN NUMBER	WEEK STARTING							WEEK STARTING						
EXERCISES COMPLETED	NO. OF SETS/REPS							NO. OF SETS-REPS						
NO. OF TIMES PROGRAM COMPLETED THIS WEEK TECHNIQUE NOTES														
NOTES ON ANY OTHER ACTIVITY														

TRAINING LOG

119

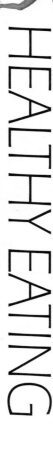

FOOD DIARY

Make a note of everything you eat and drink so that you have a constant record of the changes you make to your eating habits. Mark down your mood swings throughout the day and what you think may have caused them. This will help you determine if a particular food has led to an eating binge. Be sure also to make a note if you managed to resist temptation and pass on a piece of cake. Don't forget to make some copies of the blank log so you can continue to chart your progress.

NAME			DATE	
FOOD	AMOUNT	TIME	MOOD	GOOD JUDGEMENT

Notes (mood swings/other comments)